The International Behavioural and Social Sciences Library

T0227686

FAMILY ILL H

TAVISTOCK

FAMILIES & MARRIAGE
In 6 Volumes

FAMILY ILL HEALTH

An Investigation in General Practice

ROBERT KELLNER

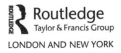

Routledge
Taylor & Francis Group

LONDON AND NEW YORK

First published in 1963 by
Tavistock Publications (1959) Limited

Published in 2001 by
Routledge
2 Park Square, Milton Park, Abingdon, Oxfordshire OX14 4RN
711 Third Avenue, New York, NY 10017

First issued in paperback 2014

Routledge is an imprint of the Taylor and Francis Group, an informa business

British Library Cataloguing in Publication Data
A CIP catalogue record for this book
is available from the British Library

Family Ill Health
ISBN 0-415-26420-0
Families & Marriage: 6 Volumes
ISBN 0-415-26508-8
The International Behavioural and Social Sciences Library
112 Volumes
ISBN 0-415-25670-4

ISBN 13: 978-1-138-87586-9 (pbk)
ISBN 13: 978-0-415-26420-4 (hbk)

Family Ill Health

An Investigation in General Practice

ROBERT KELLNER
M.B., Ch.B.

TAVISTOCK PUBLICATIONS

CHARLES C THOMAS · PUBLISHER

First published in 1963
by Tavistock Publications (1959) Limited
2 Park Square, Milton Park, Abingdon, Oxon, OX14 4RN
in 11 point Times Roman by
C. Tinling & Co. Ltd., Liverpool, London and Prescot

First published in 1963
in the United States of America
by Charles C Thomas · Publisher
301-327 East Lawrence Avenue, Springfield, Illinois

To H.A.F.

CONTENTS

LIST OF FIGURES AND TABLES

List of Figures and Tables

CASE NOTES

AN APPRECIATION

My sincere thanks to Mr M. C. K. Tweedie and Mr B. Selby of the Sub-Department of Mathematical Statistics, University of Liverpool, for preparing the report on page 105; to Dr Bertram Brooker for reading the manuscript and helpful criticism; and to my wife Dr Diana A. Kellner for her invaluable help.

R. KELLNER

March 1962

CHAPTER 1

The Plan of the Investigation

INTRODUCTION

A family doctor is concerned with the health of several members of the same family and sometimes two or more generations are under his care. He is in the position to observe the social, economic, and emotional consequences of the illness of one member on his close relatives.

Families differ in health; the stock, the childhood and home, and infection may be responsible for ill health in more than one member. Sometimes physical illness, mental illness, and social factors all play their part in making a family ill and in need of continuous support, while in other families more fortunate circumstances create a sturdy self-reliance.

What happens when one member falls ill? How does the illness affect the others? Does it influence their mood and contentment only or may it affect even their health? How does the mother's or the father's illness affect the children? This volume does not attempt to answer all these questions. Only some of the effects of illness within the family have been investigated. It is limited to a survey of families in a general practice, the illnesses are often minor ones, and the consequences seldom serious.

The patient's decision to seek his doctor's help was regarded

1

as the unit of illness; an attendance at the surgery or a request for a visit at home are items which can be counted and thus to some extent measured. Sometimes the request for help was influenced by events within the family, mostly it was not.

The idea of undertaking this survey occurred to me while I was tabulating the seasonal incidence of minor mental ill health in our general practice. The attendances were unevenly distributed and, apart from infections, which produced crops of entries on the attendance charts, there were other groupings which were unexplained. On the chart of one family there was a 'cluster' of entries, which I remembered was caused by a minor epidemic within the family; however, one of the members had what I regarded as 'functional' symptoms.

This was the actual entry in the protocol:

i

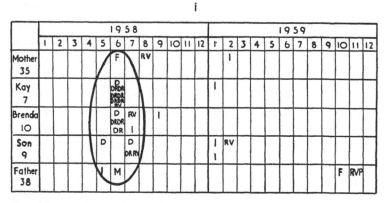

		1958												1959											
	1	2	3	4	5	6	7	8	9	10	11	12	1	2	3	4	5	6	7	8	9	10	11	12
Mother 35						F		RV						1											
Kay 7						D DRDR DRDR DRDR RV							1											
Brenda 10						D DRDR DR	RV 1	1						1											
Son 9					D	D DRRV							1 1	RV											
Father 38						M																F	RVP	

The code[1] means: F = functional. D = Domiciliary visit. R means revisit, e.g. DR domiciliary revisit, RV = Revisit at the surgery. M = Medicine a sign to indicate that the patient did not attend himself or that someone else wanted to collect a prescription for him.

On reading the case sheets and the visiting book to see what had happened I found that there were nineteen entries in June and July 1958. I had visited the home on 12 June because Kay, the younger daughter, was ill and had complained to her mother of a sore throat. When I saw her she

[1] Details of the code and method are included as Appendix I.

was restless and flushed and her mother told me that she was not eating and had been rambling at times. Her temperature was 104, pulse 120 per minute, she had slightly tender enlarged jugular lymph nodes but I could not detect other abnormal signs. She looked very ill.

The pyrexia lasted for three days and on the fourth day she had almost no residual symptoms. I have no record of what I told the mother but I probably said that I did not know the cause of the infection and that I would have to observe the child until I was certain. (On reflection, it was almost certainly a virus infection because after three days the sister and later the brother developed an almost identical illness of the same duration.)

There is no doubt that the mother was very worried by her daughter's illness. I visited the girl twice a day. She was getting neither better nor worse, and I examined her repeatedly hoping to find signs to explain the temperature. I could not fully reassure the mother because I also was worried; I wondered whether I was justified in withholding the routine investigations.

On 16 June, that is on the first day the daughter felt better, the mother came to the surgery with pruritus vulvae. She told me that she had had pruritus for seven years, but that it was never bad enough to tell a doctor about. I could not find anything abnormal on examination and thought that her symptoms were 'functional'. I decided not to investigate at that time. I told her that she had no organic illness and that she was to come back if the pruritus did not go. (I saw her at a later date and she had no symptoms.)

Four days later the mother came again and wanted a 'prescription for piles' for her husband. I asked her to tell her husband to come and see me but he did not do so. The other entries in this cluster are due to to the infection and seem of little importance.

At the time I did not associate the mother's attendance with the daughter's illness; she was one of many patients on a busy day. The mother's symptoms were mild and did not seem important; but it is interesting that, after the daughter had a worrying illness, the mother complained for the first time of pruritus although she had had it for seven years.

In psychiatric literature there are many references on emotional interactions within the family, chiefly between a young child and the mother. Balint and his collaborators (1957) described interactions in the family causing ill health and based their work on observation in general practice.

Buck and Laughton (1959) compared the illnesses of children of neurotic and those of healthy parents; they based their work on insurance records which included the services of the general practitioner. Hopkins (1959), also in general practice, described families in which 'transmission of illness' had occurred and used 'ill health charts' to demonstrate this. To my knowledge no one has attempted to investigate the incidence of this phenomenon in general practice and the incidence of the various forms it can take.

This volume is divided into three main parts and each corresponds to a stage in the survey. Chapter 2 consists of case histories of selected families in which apparently some form of interaction produced the paired entries or clusters noted on the attendance charts. In Chapter 3 the various types and causes of pairs are discussed and the roles of family members are investigated. In Chapter 4 attendance rates are investigated in order to assess whether interactions—if they occurred—affected the attendance rates of families.

THE PRACTICE AND THE PATIENTS

The practice was a partnership of two, in an area partly urban and partly semi-rural. The families were chosen from the half of the practice in which I worked, because my partner did most of the work in the other half. My part contained a branch surgery on the outskirts of a northern city and the majority of patients came from a working-class district and an adjoining industrial estate. About 250 patients lived on a small industrial estate two and a half miles away, a few families came from a near-by wealthy district, and a few others lived in the city.

We had full diagnostic facilities at the local hospitals, thus all X-ray and laboratory investigations would be performed at these departments on request by general practitioners. We had beds in a small maternity hospital where our patients were delivered. The consultant services were well organized and we were fortunate that there were only short waiting lists for outpatient clinic appointments. It is a small practice and there was time to keep adequate records.

The exact number of patients was found by checking the Executive Council's list and from replies to a sociological questionnaire which was used for another investigation. The initial survey comprised 1,735 patients. The conditions for including a patient in this study were: that the patient had been registered with us for the last two consecutive years (1958 and 1959); that he lived within a three-mile radius of the branch surgery; and that at least two members of the same family were our patients. The other patients were excluded.

The remaining patients consisted of 356 families. Close relatives living in separate households and more distant relatives living in the same household were investigated together. The majority of the families consisted of parents and their children, and sometimes one or two grandparents living in the same or in a separate household.

The records in the main surgery were checked in order not to miss the attendances of patients who on rare occasions decided to go to the more distant surgery. The records of the home visits were kept by our receptionist and I made clinical notes about these in the visiting book. At the end of two years the visits were entered on attendance charts like the one above. This code was used in the original protocol and some of the symbols are of no import in the present investigation. The following services have not been entered on the charts: immunization and vaccination, maternity work, and attendances for repeat prescriptions and for medical certificates. These services have not the same significance as those due to illness. On some charts attendances for repeat prescriptions have been entered when these appeared to be of interest but they have not been included in the attendance rates. The details of the method and the full code are included in Appendix I.

The charts have been used as illustrations because some of the attendance patterns are difficult to visualize, but they are not essential to the text.

CHAPTER 2

Case Notes

The following procedure was adopted to find families in which interaction may have occurred. All families were selected in which a member had an overt emotional disturbance or had attended with functional[1] symptoms. The details of the attendances from the case notes and from the visiting book were entered on larger charts and these were examined. The families in which interaction may have occurred were then divided into four groups, the criterion being chiefly the frequency of attendance of the family members. As this division is arbitrary there is a considerable overlap between these groups.

GROUP I. RARE ATTENDERS

The first group investigated were those families which had at least one member who attended relatively rarely. The paired entries and clusters on these charts were conspicuous and it was easier to study them because they were separate from other attendances. In twelve of these families some sort of interaction had apparently occurred. Eleven are listed below and one is described in the next chapter.

[1] The term 'functional symptom' has been used to describe all somatic symptoms which were apparently not caused by organic pathology.

No. I

	1958												1959											
	1	2	3	4	5	6	7	8	9	10	11	12	1	2	3	4	5	6	7	8	9	10	11	12
Daughter 26		CP			CP	CP	DP RVP	RVP					CP RVP RVP	CP ECT			CP			CP				
Mother 56								F																
Father 83			D																					

FAMILY 1

3 in household. Father, 83, retired solicitor. Mother, 56, housewife. Daughter, 26, unmarried, clerk.

The daughter had recurrent endogenous depressions. She attended a psychiatric outpatient clinic and also came to the surgery frequently, usually escorted by her mother.

Aug. 1958. Daughter visited at home. She was severely depressed and was admitted to a mental hospital for treatment. While she was in hospital the mother came to the surgery and complained of soreness of both breasts; I could find no abnormal signs. The mother also mentioned that she was very worried about her daughter.

May 1958. Father visited at home, when he had an upper respiratory tract infection.

The father's minor illness is not related to those of the rest of the family. The mother's only attendance seems to be directly due to the daughter's illness.

No. 2

	1958												1959											
	1	2	3	4	5	6	7	8	9	10	11	12	1	2	3	4	5	6	7	8	9	10	11	12
Daughter 27		P RVP RVP		I												I	Pregnancy							
Son 30		I																						
Father 59			I									I			I	RV								

8

FAMILY 2

3 in household. Father, widower, 59, platelayer. Daughter, 27, unmarried, shorthand typist. Son, 30, single, engineer. One single son aged 20 was away on National Service.

The father had not been to the surgery for five years, the daughter had not been for two years, and the son had not attended in the ten years he had been registered as a National Health Service patient.

11 March 1958. Daughter came to surgery and told me that she could not eat or sleep and was worrying all the time and losing weight. Her mother had died one year previously, and now in addition to her office job she had to do the housework and look after her father and her brother. I could not detect any abnormality on examination except that she looked anxious and tense. Her chest X-ray and urine were normal. She re-attended twice.

19 March. Son attended with acne vulgaris which he had been scratching, and asked me for treatment for his skin.

26 April. Father attended, with a mild upper respiratory tract infection.

June. Daughter attended with spasmodic dysmenorrhoea. She was married in November, and moved into her new home.

Dec. Father attended and complained of difficulty in reading. He was found to be presbyopic and was referred to an optician.

1 April 1959. Father attended with bronchitis.

9 April. Daughter came complaining of indigestion.

In March and April 1958 three members of this family attended within a short period. The son apparently started to scratch his face at the same time that his sister had an anxiety state. He attended eight days after his sister's first visit although he had not made a single attendance for at least ten years and he has not attended since. The father's visit could have been a coincidence, but it is possible that during the previous five years he had had similar minor ailments and taken them in his stride. The other attendances do not appear to be of importance.

No. 3

	1958												1959											
	1	2	3	4	5	6	7	8	9	10	11	12	1	2	3	4	5	6	7	8	9	10	11	12
Mother 42	I												?											
Charles 10													F											
Peter 18											F		I RV											
Arthur 21						I	RV RV	P	RVP	RVP	RVP		P											

FAMILY 3

5 in household. Father, 46, railwayman. Mother, 42, house-wife. Three sons, Arthur, 21, coal porter. Peter, 18, apprentice. Charles, 10, schoolboy. The father is on another general practitioner's list.

Apart from one attendance in February 1958, the mother had not been for over three years. Similarly, Charles had not been for over three years, and Peter not for eleven years.

Feb. 1958. Mother attended with mild bronchitis.

May. Arthur was involved in a road accident. He was hit by a car while cycling. He was concussed, fractured his skull, and had a lower motor neurone lesion of his left facial nerve. He was discharged from the hospital at the end of June, but he attended the surgical outpatient clinic and also the Physiotherapy Department.

I saw him first after his discharge from hospital. He attended again in July complaining of severe headaches. Later he became depressed, probably partly because of the facial palsy. He said on one occasion: 'I wish the chap had killed me instead of leaving me like this.' He re-attended once a month; he had symptoms which appeared to be func-

10

tional and were related to the left side of his face and head. In August there were slight movements of the orbicularis oculi and the function of his facial muscles continued to improve. Eventually he made a complete recovery.

13 Nov. Peter attended complaining of a sore throat 'first thing each morning' accompanied by a headache and said that both symptoms passed off quickly. I detected no abnormalities on examination.

1 Jan. 1959. Shortly after midnight I was called to their home. Arthur had been drinking on New Year's Eve and after returning home became violent. He had attacked his father, broken Charles's new toys, broken windows, and smashed pieces of furniture. While I was in the house he was excited and aggressive and tried to attack his father again. After about an hour he became somewhat quieter and I managed to persuade him to come with me to the mental hospital and to stay there as a voluntary patient. He took his own discharge two days later.

21 Jan. Mother came with Charles to the surgery. She told me that she had a 'bilious attack', and she 'felt sick', and that she had vomited. She also told me that Charles was 'off colour', and he 'did not eat' and that he 'grinds his teeth' at night. I could not detect any abnormal signs.

12 Feb. Peter came to the surgery. He had been seen a week previously by my partner, whose note reads: 'laryngitis'. When I saw him he appeared well.

Peter had not needed a doctor for eleven years; his first attendance after this interval complaining of functional symptoms coincides with his brother's 'traumatic neurosis'. He had a minor organic illness in February but it is doubtful whether he would have felt the need to come to the surgery in the normal course of events. At the time of writing—March 1961—i.e. thirteen years after his mother registered him as a National Health Service patient, his only two attendances have been at the time of his brother's distress.

11

Charles had not been to the surgery for over three years. He witnessed his brother's violence and appeared to be terrified when I visited their home on that occasion. It is therefore very likely that his minor emotional disturbance was due to this experience and to the tension in the home.

The mother's first attendance in three years in February 1958 appears to be unimportant. Her 'bilious attack' in January 1959 could have been an organic condition—a minor 'gastritis'—but it is more likely that it was caused by anxiety because the previous entry in her case notes in 1955 reads: ' "bilious attack". Very anxious and tense.'

This case is, in some ways, similar to the preceding one. Here also, a long spell of good health was interrupted by the illness and unhappiness of one member of the family.

No. 4

	1958												1959											
	1	2	3	4	5	6	7	8	9	10	11	12	1	2	3	4	5	6	7	8	9	10	11	12
Wife 39									P	Pr	Pr													
Husband 43		I						I	P				I RV										Rec	

FAMILY 4

3 in household. Husband, 43, fitter. Wife, 39, shop-assistant. Son, 19, fitter.

March 1958. Husband attended complaining of deafness. He was found to have wax in both ears.

14 July. Husband attended because of a swollen elbow. He was found to have a distended right olecranon bursa.

26 Aug. Wife complained that she was 'obsessed with what people were talking about' that she 'had to listen to what they were saying', that she was 'all on edge', that she 'got worked up', and that it made her 'sick'. She re-attended twice for repeat prescriptions.

28 Aug. Husband attended complaining that his 'nerves

12

were bad'. He also complained of a sore anus but refused examination.

Jan. 1959. Husband attended complaining of rectal bleeding; this was later found to be due to internal haemorrhoids. He revisited once, and had a recurrence in November.

Two days after the wife first attended because of her minor neurotic illness, the husband attended, and this was the only time that he complained of 'bad nerves'. The other entries are not relevant.

No. 5

	1958												1959											
	1	2	3	4	5	6	7	8	9	10	11	12	1	2	3	4	5	6	7	8	9	10	11	12
Mother 55		I RV		D DR		Rec	RV RVRV							I				Rec	RV					
Daughter 15						F																		

FAMILY 5
2 in household. Mother, 55, schoolteacher. Daughter, 15, schoolgirl. One son, 13, is away at a boarding-school.
Feb. 1958. Mother attended with a mild gastritis.
25 April. Mother seen at home. She had urticaria of the eyelids, the forehead, and the neck. The eyelids were the most affected and were swollen. I did not know the cause of the urticaria and therefore treated her symptomatically with oral antihistamines.
30 June. Mother came to the surgery with daughter. The mother had a recurrence of the urticaria involving the eyelids, and the conjunctivae were hyperaemic. She also told me that the daughter was blinking excessively. I found that the girl had a habit spasm, she screwed up her eyes frequently, and was also, in fact, blinking excessively. I could find no organic cause.
July. Mother attended with a painful osteoarthritic knee, and re-attended three times.

Feb. 1959. Mother had bronchitis followed by a recurrence in May.

The daughter's only attendance was for a functional disorder. Her behaviour vaguely imitated that of her mother, and the onset coincided with the mother's first urticaria. It is possible that the mother's complaint started the daughter's habit.

No. 6

	19 58.												1959											
	1	2	3	4	5	6	7	8	9	10	11	12	1	2	3	4	5	6	7	8	9	10	11	12
Mother 49													F						F RVP					
Father 50												I												
Son 17													I	RV										
Daughter 10																	I							

FAMILY 6

4 in household. Father, 50, railwayman. Mother, 49, housewife. Son, 17, factory worker. Daughter, 10, schoolgirl.

The father, mother, and daughter had not been to the surgery for three years and the son had not attended for seven years.

6 Dec. 1958. Father attended, complaining of excessive thirst, frequency of micturition, and loss of weight. I found no abnormality on physical examination, but the Benedict test showed a large amount of sugar in the urine. I told him that he was diabetic and would need continuous treatment, and referred him to a diabetic clinic.

23 Jan. 1959. Mother attended complaining that she had 'no appetite' and that she felt tired. When I asked for further details about her symptoms she told me that she had been tired 'for the last two years'. I could not detect any abnormalities on examination.

29 Feb. Son attended with an upper respiratory tract infection, and he told me that his nose bled each time he had a head cold.

May. Daughter attended, with pharyngitis.

July. Mother re-attended with a recurrence of functional symptoms.

First the father became a regular attender at the surgery for prescriptions for insulin, testing reagents, needles, etc. Next the mother attended with a functional complaint which she had had for two years. Then the son, who had not attended for seven years, came complaining of nose bleeds which he had had previously. It seems that both delayed their visit to the surgery until the father started to attend. The daughter's minor illness may have been a coincidence.

No. 7

		1958												1959										
	1	2	3	4	5	6	7	8	9	10	11	12	1	2	3	4	5	6	7	8	9	10	11	12
Daughter 20							I	Rec	Rec			Rec									D DR DR			
Mother 54																					P	RVP		

FAMILY 7

3 in household. Family of 4. Father, 58, civil servant. Mother, 54, housewife. Daughter, 20, schoolteacher, unmarried. Son, 24, businessman. The father is on another general practitioner's list. The son spends part of the year away from home.

July 1958. Daughter attended with spasmodic dysmenorrhoea and re-attended three times with the same complaint.

2 Sept. 1959. Daughter visited at home and found to have glandular fever. She was revisited at home and later seen by my partner before returning to work.

5 Sept. Mother attended with symptoms and signs of an anxiety state.

Oct. Mother re-attended, she had improved considerably.

The mother's anxiety state, and her only attendance, occurred three days later after her daughter became ill. When I saw the daughter at home I told the mother that the illness was not serious and the mother had no cause for anxiety. It is interesting that the mother's reaction (if it was due to the daughter's illness) was out of proportion to the minor stress.

No. 8

							1958										1959						
	1	2	3	4	5	6	7	8	9	10	11	12	1	2	3	4	5	6	7	8	9	10	11	12
Sister 20		I	RV RV		I																			
Brother 16			F								I F													

FAMILY 8

4 in household. Sister, 20, unmarried, shorthand typist. Brother, 16, apprentice. The father and mother are on another general practitioner's list.

The sister had not attended for two years, and the brother not for three years.

24 Feb. Sister attended with urticaria on both hands. I could not find an allergen and decided to treat her symptomatically with oral antihistamines. She re-attended 3 March.

25 March. Sister came to surgery with brother, who complained of a dull ache in both loins. He told me that he had spells of this ache lasting for two weeks and that these had started two years previously. He said that the pain was not severe and that he could feel it only at night in bed. He looked well and I could not detect any abnormalities on examination.

May. Sister had a mild upper respiratory tract infection.

Oct. Brother had laryngitis and also a recurrence of his backache. The history was similar; again I detected no

16

abnormality and reassured him that the ache was not due to an organic illness. He had no further recurrence of his symptoms.

After three years the brother's first attendance coincided with the sister's minor ailment. As with case 7, the brother delayed coming to the surgery until his sister had started to attend.

No. 9

	1958												1959											
	1	2	3	4	5	6	7	8	9	10	11	12	1	2	3	4	5	6	7	8	9	10	11	12
Mother 38																I								
Daughter 13																	DF DF	F						

FAMILY 9
3 in household. Father, 41, shop manager. Mother, 38, housewife. Daughter, 13, at a grammar school.
    The mother had not been to the surgery for six years and the daughter not for four years.
15 April. Mother attended complaining of one episode of severe headache. She gave a typical description of an attack of migraine.
2 May. Daughter seen at home by my partner; she was complaining of abdominal pain. He found no abnormal signs.
28 May. Daughter seen again at home by my partner, with a recurrence of the abdominal pain. Again he found no evidence of organic illness.
13 June. Daughter attended surgery with mother. She told me that 'it was not really a pain, but a tumbling-over of the stomach'; she 'felt sickly with it' and it was 'like an avalanche'. I could not detect any abnormality on examination; I reassured the mother and daughter that there was

17

no cause for anxiety and that these sensations were not due to an organic illness.

Although they had not needed a doctor for six and four years respectively, the mother and daughter had illnesses which occurred within 16 days of each other.

Follow-up: I saw the girl again in May 1960. She came with her mother to the surgery and this time she complained about 'sickly feelings' which lasted for about one hour and made her 'double up'. The mother had tried many remedies including analgesics and various alkalies, and the only one which seemed to help was a proprietary preparation containing salicylates and sodium bicarbonate. I asked the mother if I could have a talk with the daughter alone and I took a more detailed history. She appeared to be a happy, well-mannered child, and did not seem to be anxious or tense. She did not admit to any worries except that she had a 'crush on a boy' and also there were two 'rough girls in the neighbourhood' who used to abuse her when they met her in the street.

I questioned her again about her discomfort, and she told me that she usually had it when she came home after school games. She very rarely had the discomfort away from home, if she had it, it was not severe and lasted 'only half an hour or so'. She never had symptoms when she was on holidays, nor when she was with other girls, nor could she remember having it when her mother was away from home. The mother was devoted to her only child and the girl spent most of her free time with her.

I gave her two tablets of amylobarbiton gr.¾., advised her to take one when she had the 'sickly feeling', and told her to come and see me again in two weeks' time. On their next attendance the daughter told me that the tablet had 'completely taken the feeling away'. While they were both in the surgery I mentioned to them that it seemed that the

18

daughter had the discomfort only when she was with her mother. 'This is not very flattering for me, is it?' the mother asked. I reassured her that it was not her fault, and tried to hint that this might not have happened had her emotions been less intense. On the next visit the daughter was symptom-free and she has not had abdominal discomfort since.

When I first saw the daughter I did not suspect the cause of her symptoms and I only reassured her and the mother. I did not even take a full history, partly because I regarded the symptoms as trivial, partly because, in general practice, one has to allot one's time according to the apparent needs of the case, and can provide psychotherapy for only a few patients. Therefore functional symptoms are often treated by reassurance only.

Wolff (1952), and Hunter and Ross (1960) have demonstrated the emotional factors in the aetiology of migraine, and it is interesting that the daughter's functional symptoms were preceded by the mother's solitary attack of migraine.

Because the second episode throws some light on the origin of the cluster I felt justified in describing it in detail. It seems that the mother's and daughter's illnesses were due to some minor crisis in their relationship.

No. 10

	1958												1959											
	1	2	3	4	5	6	7	8	9	10	11	12	1	2	3	4	5	6	7	8	9	10	11	12
Wife 51				I	RV	S RT			RV				RV	P	RV			RV			F RVP RVP			
Husband 52											P	RVP I Pr												

The symbols in June mean S = stress, RT = radiotherapy.

FAMILY 10
2 in household. Husband, 52, clerk. Wife, 51, housewife. They have two grown-up children who live away from home.

19

The husband had not been to the surgery for over two years.

April 1958. Wife attended with upper respiratory tract infection.

May. She re-attended, and was found to have a hard lump in her left breast and hard lymph glands in the axilla. She was referred to a surgical outpatient clinic, and from there admitted for biopsy. The histiological section showed an anaplastic carcinoma.

4 June. She attended, complaining that she felt tense. At that time she was waiting for the result of a chest X-ray. The same month she had a course of pre-operative radiotherapy.

Sept. She attended because the biopsy wound would not heal. She was admitted on 17 November to a surgical ward for a simple mastectomy and excision of axillary glands and was discharged on 17 January.

Nov. Husband attended the surgery after the wife had been admitted; he complained of feeling depressed. He was seen by my partner who gave him a prescription for a preparation containing dexamphetamine.

3 Dec. Husband re-attended, still complaining of depression.

8 Dec. Husband attended and told me he had a head cold.

10 Dec. He re-attended and asked for a repeat prescription of the tablets.

After her discharge from hospital I saw the wife on seven occasions. On three of these she attended because of pain in the scar region and later she complained of headaches which I thought were functional.

The husband's depression was apparently reactive; after not having been to the surgery for two years, he attended three times within one week and one of these attendances was because of a head cold. It is likely that he would have ignored this minor illness had he not been lonely and unhappy.

No. 11

	1958												1959											
	1	2	3	4	5	6	7	8	9	10	11	12	1	2	3	4	5	6	7	8	9	10	11	12
Husband 50		I RV				Rec I															P	I	RV	
Wife 44																				P RVP RVP				

FAMILY 11

3 in household. Husband, 50, clerk. Wife, 44, housewife. Son, 9, schoolboy.

March 1958. Husband attended with conjunctivitis, and re-attended once.

June 1958. Husband attended with recurrence of con-junctivitis and also had acne rosacea. He re-attended three days later.

15 Aug. 1959. Wife came to the surgery and said that she was depressed and afraid. She also reported dreaming repeatedly that she was shop-lifting.

18 Aug. She re-attended with the same complaint. She was apprehended a few days later by the police, having in fact stolen a small item in a shop.

24 Aug. Wife re-attended, greatly distressed, and my partner referred her to a psychiatric outpatient clinic.

3 Sept. Husband attended and complained that he felt 'jittery'. He was anxious because his wife was awaiting proceedings on the shop-lifting charge. (The consultant psychiatrist, my partner, and I tried to find a way to save her from going to court, but she had to appear before the magistrate. She was bound over for one year.)

11 Oct. Husband attended with bronchial asthma.

10 Nov. He re-attended because his broncho-spasm was still persisting.

It is interesting that the wife's apparently compulsive action was preceded by dreams that predicted the deed. The wife's illness seemed to have precipitated a mild anxiety state,

C 21

and later a psychosomatic illness in the husband, though this may have been partly due to worry over the legal proceedings.

GROUP II. AVERAGE ATTENDERS

The investigation of families of average attenders was more difficult. The members of these families attended more often than those described in the previous group and many of the attendances were for minor ailments. Therefore paired entries and clusters occurred more frequently; in many of them it was doubtful whether interaction had occurred and in others the paired entries were almost certainly coincidental. Nine of these families are listed below.[1]

No. 12

	1958												1959											
	1	2	3	4	5	6	7	8	9	10	11	12	1	2	3	4	5	6	7	8	9	10	11	12
Mother 39							FO RVP RVP	P RVP	I	I DR RV				I										
Daughter 12									I					I				P			I			
Father 46								D			D													
Son 9													P						F					

FAMILY 12

4 in household. Father, 46, paint-mixer. Mother, 39, house-wife. Daughter, 12; son, 9, both at school.

The father is an epileptic, and takes anti-convulsant drugs regularly.

13 July. Wife came to the surgery. She had a small wound near an old osteomyelitis scar and she complained of pain in the left patella and that she felt 'trembly' and could not sleep.

17 July. Wife re-attended; the wound was slightly infected but she felt less tense since taking sedatives.

21 July. Further re-attendance of wife.

1 Aug. Father attempted suicide by taking an overdose of

[1] One family has been described in the introduction.

barbiturates and anti-convulsants and was admitted to a mental hospital. He was discharged on 3 September.

11 Aug. Wife attended, now with a severe anxiety state.

12 Aug. Wife re-attended.

3 Sept. Wife attended and complained that some of her anxiety symptoms had returned prior to her menses.

13 Sept. Daughter attended complaining that her arm was 'sore' after a diphtheria immunization undergone two days previously. On examination, there was slight tenderness only, at the site of the injection.

14 Sept. Mother attended with a mild laryngitis.

13 Oct. Mother visited at home; she had cystitis and after treatment for five days re-attended once.

21 Nov. Husband again attempted suicide by taking an overdose of phenobarbitone and was again admitted to a mental hospital (he was discharged on 7 February).

1 Jan. Mother came with the son. She complained that he was very restless at night.

21 March. Daughter had a very mild bronchitis.

28 March. Mother attended with a contact eczema due to a deodorant.

12 July. Daughter attended and told me that she was 'worried all the time', that she could not sleep and that she woke up at six o'clock in the morning. 'I worry a tremendous lot even about the slightest little thing, for instance, when Mummy is a little bit late.' She was a nail-biter and had a habit-spasm of wrinkling her nose and distorting her mouth. I referred her to a child psychiatrist.

Oct. Daughter had a mild upper respiratory tract infection.

Oct. Mother came with son, and told me that the boy had had a few attacks of 'flu' and that he was losing weight. I could detect no abnormality on examination.

The husband's first suicidal attempt was preceded by the wife's mild anxiety symptoms; followed by her mental state becoming worse. Her reaction after her husband was admitted to a mental hospital is understandable; it is also possible that some tension in the family preceded the husband's suicidal attempt and that the wife's initial symptoms were due to the same stress.

After the wife's first attendance in July there followed a period of ill health in the family and (apart from her cystitis, which was probably coincidental, though this is discussed below) it is possible that their distress was partly responsible for these other attendances.

The father's second attempted suicide was not reflected in subsequent family ill health except for the son's mild symptoms while the father was in hospital. The daughter's emotional disturbance does not take part in a cluster on the attendance chart; she was a nervous child, and her symptoms were probably aggravated by the tension in the home.

No. 13

	1958												1959											
	1	2	3	4	5	6	7	8	9	10	11	12	1	2	3	4	5	6	7	8	9	10	11	12
Father 31											F	F F								I				
Mother 27											F	F												
Carol 4									D DRDR	I	I RV							D				I		
Alma 2																		D DR						

FAMILY 13

4 in household. Father, 31, clerk. Mother, 27, part-time secretary. Two girls, Carol, 4, Alma, 2.

26 Aug. Carol seen at home. She had a right-sided pyelitis, and I treated her with sulphonamides.

18 Sept. Mother attended, and said that she had been losing weight for the last month. I could not detect any abnormal signs on examination. Her chest X-ray was normal, her urine, E.S.R., and full blood count were within normal limits.

25 Sept. Mother came to surgery with Carol and complained about the girl's scalp; she had mild dandruff.

2 Oct. Mother re-attended having lost another 3 lb. I asked her to keep a weight chart and to re-attend in a month's time if she had lost further weight.

27 Oct. Mother brought Carol to surgery, with a mild upper respiratory tract infection. Her own weight was stationary.

31 Oct. Mother and Carol re-attended; Carol's cough had now subsided.

7 Nov. Father attended complaining of headache. I detected no abnormality on examination and tried to reassure him.

21 Nov. Father re-attended and complained that he felt 'sleepy all the time'.

28 Nov. Father re-attended, he was seen by my partner whose entry reads 'multiple psychosomatic symptoms. Says: the wife does not want another child.'

19 June 1959. Carol had recurrence of pyelitis. She had a high temperature, was in severe pain and was admitted to hospital for treatment. She was discharged on 11 July.

29 July. Alma seen at home, with mild bronchitis.

11 Sept. Father had contact dermatitis on both hands.

9 Oct. Carol had a mild upper respiratory tract infection.

Carol's mild pyelitis in August probably does not belong to the cluster because it does not appear to have been the 'precipitating illness'. The mother's loss of weight and the father's mild neurotic illness were probably due to some marital tension. Carol's three attendances at the time of this minor family crisis might have been coincidental, but it could be that during this period the mother was less able to cope with the child's ailments.

No. 14

	1958												1959											
	1	2	3	4	5	6	7	8	9	10	11	12	1	2	3	4	5	6	7	8	9	10	11	12
Wife 36								F		///// ///// Pregnancy ///// /////			I									I	RV	
																						I		
Husband 34			F					?	F	RVP											DF P RVP RVP	I RVP		

FAMILY 14

6 in household. Father, 34, labourer. Mother, 36, housewife. Three daughters, 12, 8, 5. One son, 9.

March 1958. Husband attended and complained of muscular pains. I could detect no abnormality on examination.

26 Aug. Husband re-attended and complained of vague abdominal pains. I could not find any abnormality but I was not certain of the diagnosis. I asked him to come again or to call me if he did not feel better.

30 Aug. Wife came to surgery. She complained of headaches and told me that they were not relieved by the analgesics she had taken. I could not find any organic cause and I gave her a few tablets of amylobarbitone grn.¾. advising her to take one the next time she had the headache. I also asked her to come again but she did not re-attend.

26 Sept. Husband attended and complained of recurrent headaches. The description was strongly suggestive of a functional origin to his symptoms. I could find no abnormality on examination.

6 Oct. Husband re-attended with the same complaint, and I tried to reassure him that his headaches were not due to an organic illness.

The wife had an uncomplicated pregnancy from September 1958 till June 1959. She had a trichomonas vaginitis in January 1959.

10 Sept. 1959. Husband seen at home. He complained of 'muscle stiffness' which had started a few days previously and which was not caused by unusual muscular exertion. He looked well, his pulse and temperature were normal, and I found nothing abnormal on physical examination.

20 Sept. Husband attended with a variety of hypochondriacal symptoms.

20-27 Sept. Husband re-attended twice.

2 Oct. Husband attended complaining of cough. He had a mild upper respiratory tract infection.

10 Oct. Wife attended with a recurrence of the trichomonas vaginitis and she also complained of low backache. This was apparently due to a mobile retroversion of the uterus, the pain was relieved when the position of the uterus was corrected and recurred when the Hodge pessary slipped and the uterus retroverted.

29 Oct. Husband attended with a recurrence of his hypochondriasis.

Nov. Wife attended for reinsertion of the pessary.

In August 1958 the wife's functional headaches coincided with the husband's minor neurotic illness. In September and October 1959 the wife's attendances followed those of her husband, but hers were due to organic causes and therefore this cluster of attendances is probably coincidental.

No. 15

	1958												1959											
	1	2	3	4	5	6	7	8	9	10	11	12	1	2	3	4	5	6	7	8	9	10	11	12
Grand-mother 55	CO					P										RV	RV	RV						1
Grand-father 56				D RV / DDR	RV FO RV/RV																			
Grand-daughter 6				1	DR. RV							1					F							1

FAMILY 15

4 in household. Grandfather, 56, factory security officer. Grandmother, 55, housewife. Granddaughter, 6. The granddaughter is an illegitimate child, and lives with the grandparents. Her mother lives in another city.

Feb. 1958. Grandmother attended for treatment of chronic seborrhoeic dermatitis.

2 April. Grandfather visited at home. He had influenza.

7 April. Grandfather attended surgery.

23 April. Granddaughter visited at home. She had an upper respiratory tract infection.

29 April. Grandmother brought granddaughter to surgery with an otitis media.

30 April. Grandfather visited at home, he had a severe low backache and symptoms and signs of an intervertebral disc protrusion, but the pain improved after a few days of bed rest. After getting up he continued to improve, and repeatedly revisited the surgery until the end of May, when he returned to work.

9 May. Grandfather attended complaining of vague abdominal pain, but I could detect no abnormality on examination.

26 June. Grandmother came to surgery with granddaughter. The child had a purulent tonsillitis with cervical lymphadenitis. The grandmother told me that she had had three 'attacks of dizziness, of feeling faint and shaky' during the last three weeks, I detected no abnormal signs, apart from noticing that she looked tense and anxious.

27 June. Granddaughter revisited at home.

30 June. Granddaughter attended surgery for re-inspection.

April 1959. Grandmother attended surgery. She had severe eczema of both hands and forearms, which responded only slowly to treatment.

May, and 27 June. Grandmother re-attended, by which time her skin was almost normal.

30 June. Grandmother attended with granddaughter and told me that the child had abdominal pain and also pain in her right shoulder. The child looked well and I could not detect any abnormality on examination.

Dec. Both granddaughter and grandmother had upper respiratory tract infections.

There was a period of ill health in the family from April till June 1958. This cluster seems to be of little significance, except for the grandmother's functional symptoms which followed her husband's illness. In June 1959 the granddaughter complained of pains for which I could not find an organic cause. These occurred after the grandmother's distressing dermatitis. There were only two occasions on which the grandmother and granddaughter complained of symptoms that were apparently of emotional origin. In each case these were preceded by the illness of another member of the family.

No. 16

	1958												1959											
	1	2	3	4	5	6	7	8	9	10	11	12	1	2	3	4	5	6	7	8	9	10	11	12
Mother 42									1															
Jennifer 16 (Step-daughter)									1															
Mary 14			1						1			1									1		P	
Carol 16						1			1 RV			1					D DR DR D				1 RV RV			

FAMILY 16

5 in household. Father, 46, clerk. Mother, 42, shop-assistant. Mother's two daughters from her previous marriage, Carol, 16, shop-assistant, Mary, 14, schoolgirl. Father's daughter from his previous marriage, Jennifer, 16, shorthand typist.

The mother had not attended previously. Jennifer had not attended for five years. The father did not attend the surgery during the two years of this survey.

April 1958. Mary had pharyngitis.

June. Carol had a mild upper respiratory tract infection.

1 Sept. Jennifer attended surgery with multiple warts on one hand.

11 Sept. Mother attended and complained that her eyes were 'sore'; she was myopic and I referred her to an optician.

15 Sept. Mary attended with a mild pharyngitis.

17 Sept. Carol attended. She had a small swelling over the root of the left lower canine. This subsided without treatment after one week.

Dec. Mary and Carol both had upper respiratory tract infections.

April 1959. Carol had a severe gastritis and needed intramuscular promazine to arrest the vomiting.

3 Sept. Carol attended surgery and told me that she had

29

lost weight. I could not detect any abnormality on examination. The miniature chest X-ray showed a suspicious shadow and the repeat film 20 September showed tuberculous shadowing of the right upper lobe. I referred her to a chest clinic.

28 Sept. Mary attended surgery with aphtous stomatitis.

19 Oct. Carol was admitted to a hospital for treatment.

29 Nov. Mary and mother attended surgery. The mother told me that Mary was 'restless and tense' and that she was losing weight. I could find nothing abnormal on examination. Her recent chest X-ray had been normal and the results of investigations were within normal limits.

There is a cluster in September 1958. With the exception of the mother, who had never visited the surgery previously, the attendances of the other members of the family are probably coincidental. Jennifer's attendance may have acted as a reminder to the mother to seek advice about her own eye discomfort, but this is uncertain.

Sircus (1959) has described cases of aphtous stomatitis in which stress appeared to be an aetiological factor. Mary, who was very attached to Carol, had aphtous stomatitis for the first time one week after her sister was told that she had tuberculosis; her only overt emotional disturbance was at the time Carol was in hospital.

No. 17

	1958												1959											
	1	2	3	4	5	6	7	8	9	10	11	12	1	2	3	4	5	6	7	8	9	10	11	12
Mother 32	I									P														
Sarah 9										D RV				DBR						I				
Reginald 12														I	I					I				
George 7					I				?		?								I					
Father 33										I RV														

30

FAMILY 17

5 in household. Father, 33, aircraft fitter. Mother, 32, housewife. Three children, Reginald, 12; Sarah, 9; George, 7.

Jan. 1958. Mother had a mild upper respiratory tract infection.

June. Mother brought George to surgery with mild bronchitis.

1 Sept. Mother came with George to surgery and told me that he had a 'stiff leg'. There was no history of injury. I could find no abnormality on examination and there was nothing to bear out the mother's observation. As I was not certain at the time about the diagnosis, I asked her to bring him back if she noticed anything unusual.

7 Oct. Sarah seen at home; she had tonsillitis.

12 Oct. Sarah re-attended surgery.

9 Oct. Father attended surgery. He had a large boil on his left hand which had caused a cellulitis.

14 Oct. Father re-attended surgery when the infection had subsided following treatment.

15 Oct. Mother came to surgery. She told me that she was 'worried about the children at night' and that she 'kept thinking that they may die'.

5 Nov. Mother brought George to surgery and told me that he 'could not walk'. I could find nothing abnormal on examination.

11 Feb. 1959. Mother attended with Reginald, he had a mild bronchitis.

25 Feb. Sarah visited at home. The mother told me that she had been 'hot' during the night and that she had complained of headache and left earache. When I examined her the left ear was discharging, she had no pain, and her temperature was normal. I revisited her on the following day. On the third day her temperature was 104, she had severe headache, photophobia, and a marked neck-stiffness, although the ear had been discharging and she had been feeling quite well on the previous day. She was admitted to

31

hospital and the lumbar puncture confirmed a purulent meningitis.

2 March. Mother brought Reginald to surgery. He had an abscess and two styes. Sarah was discharged from hospital on 10 March.

June. George had a mild upper respiratory tract infection.

Aug. Sarah had pharyngitis and Reginald had otitis media.

In October 1958 the mother had symptoms of a minor mental illness immediately after her daughter's and husband's ailments. The mother was the third member of the family to attend within six days. I have no records of how long she had had the obsessional thought that the children 'may die'. It is interesting that she complained about George's leg six weeks before her own attendance and also three weeks after. It is likely that the mother's anxiety came first and that the daughter's and husband's minor illnesses made her more anxious. It is also interesting that when Sarah had meningitis and the mother had a real cause to be worried, she weathered the storm well.

No. 18

					1958													1959							
	1	2	3	4	5	6	7	8	9	IO	II	12	1	2	3	4	5	6	7	8	9	IO	II	12
Wife 53			I																		DP	F RVP RVP	F	F
Husband 54			F	RVP RVP																				

FAMILY 18

3 in household. Husband, 54, shopkeeper. Wife, 53, housewife. Son, 24, clerk.

The husband had not been for one year. Son did not attend surgery during the two years in which the survey was carried out.

15 March 1958. Wife came to surgery. She was seen by my partner and there is only a brief entry in the case notes which reads: 'climacteric'. As he had prescribed a preparation containing stilboestrol, I assume that she had complained of 'hot flushes'.

18 March. Husband attended. He complained of feeling tired. No abnormality was found on examination. He re-attended twice in April.

Sept. 1959. Wife seen at home. She complained of feeling tired and had a variety of symptoms that were due to an anxiety neurosis; she attended five times in the course of three months.

Although the husband had not been to the surgery for over a year he came complaining of tiredness three days after his wife had 'climacteric' symptoms. However, he did not attend once in the period of four months during which his wife had a neurotic illness.

No. 19

	1958												1959											
	1	2	3	4	5	6	7	8	9	10	11	12	1	2	3	4	5	6	7	8	9	10	11	12
Mother 47	I							CO					CO					F F / F RVP						
Wilma 15																I		I / F						
Lilian 13							I																	

FAMILY 19

3 in household. Mother, 47, widow, housewife. Two daughters: Wilma, 15, shop-assistant; Lilian, 13, schoolgirl.

The mother had a congenital scoliosis and severe osteoarthritis of the spine.

Jan. 1958. Mother attended with a mild upper respiratory tract infection.

Aug. Mother and Lilian attended together. The mother had an exacerbation of her arthritis, and Lilian a mild bronchitis.

Jan. 1959. Mother re-attended with backache.

33

March. Wilma came with mother, with symptoms of pre-menstrual tension.

1 June. Wilma came with mother because of primary spasmodic dysmenorrhoea.

22 June. Mother attended complaining of feeling 'tired and listless'. I detected no abnormality on examination.

26 June. Mother re-attended, with various sensations which appeared to be functional.

20 July. Mother attended and complained of loss of appetite.

29 July. Wilma attended complaining that she had headaches every day. The headaches were not limited to the premenstrual period. I found nothing abnormal on examination.

30 July. Mother attended for a repeat prescription for sedatives and also complained of constipation.

Wilma's attendance with spasmodic dysmenorrhoea and her single attendance because of headaches were both at the time when her mother had a mild neurotic illness.

No. 20

		1958												1959											
		1	2	3	4	5	6	7	8	9	10	11	12	1	2	3	4	5	6	7	8	9	10	11	12
Mother 31		P														I	RV			Rec RV RV RV	Rec RV				
Son 8	D DR DRDR DRDR RV		RV	D DR									D DR DRDR DRDR DR	RV			DDR DRDR		I				1 RV 1	

FAMILY 20

3 in household. Father, 39, petrol-pump attendant. Mother, 31, part-time shop-assistant. Son, 8, schoolboy. The father is on another general practitioner's list.

Jan. 1958. Son visited several times at home with broncho-pneumonia.

24 Jan. Mother came with boy to the surgery for his last examination. He had no residual signs when I had seen him a week previously at home. I told the mother that he was quite fit and that he could return to school and play games, and that I would like to see him again in one month's time.

3 Feb. Mother attended and complained that she was 'all tense' and 'could not relax'.

Dec. 1958. Son had a second attack of pneumonia and again I treated him at home.

July-Oct. 1959. Mother had a tenosynovitis stenosans and was admitted to hospital in October for an operation. The other attendances on this chart were for minor ailments.

The mother's only attendance with symptoms of tension followed her son's illness, yet when the boy had pneumonia again a year later it did not seem to affect her. In view of the larger number of attendances this family could equally well have been included in the next group.

GROUP III. FREQUENT ATTENDERS

This is a mixed group and the majority of the selected families belong here. It contains chiefly families in which one or more members attended frequently and some others were included in which the cause of pairing was doubtful. Most of the pairs and clusters which may have been due to interactions were selected from a background of other attendances. The attendance charts are similar to that of family 20 and to those of Group IV.

Thirty-one of these families were found; the clusters and paired entries of ten of them are described in Appendix II (pp. 85–93).

GROUP IV. THE UNEVEN PATTERN

This group is similar to the last one in that the patients attend frequently, but in these families changes in the attendance

35

habits of two or more members occurred together. Only a summary is given here because the number of attendances is large; the individual attendances have been described in Appendix II (pp. 93–101).

Seven families were found to belong to this group and four of them are described.

No. 31

	1958												1959											
	1	2	3	4	5	6	7	8	9	10	11	12	1	2	3	4	5	6	7	8	9	10	11	12
Wife 50		F F	P F	F RVP					P		P	RVP	P ?											
Husband 48	I	I	I	F					D DR DR DR		I		II RV RV RV	RV RV									

FAMILY 31

5 in household. Husband, 48, lorry driver. Wife, 50, housewife. Three daughters, and one son, 25. Two married daughters live in separate households. One married daughter, 22, her husband, and the single son live in the household with the parents. All were our patients, except for one married daughter who lives in another part of the country.

The husband has severe lumbar osteoarthritis and wears a lumbar support. The wife frequently has minor neurotic symptoms. The other members attend rarely.

Feb.-May 1958. Husband attended with finger infections twice, and with herpes labialis once.

Sept. Husband had severe backache caused by osteoarthritis and was unable to work for a month.

Jan.-Feb. 1959. Husband had an intervertebral disc protrusion and was again off work for almost two months.

Feb. 1958-Feb. 1959. Wife had minor hypochondriacal and emotional symptoms which occurred intermittently. After February 1959 they ceased and so did the attendances of her husband (see attendance chart).

The husband was still taking salicilates regularly to relieve his pain, and the prescriptions were usually collected by his wife. Yet she did not once complain about herself during this period. The entries of the individual attendances also show that at times when the husband was most distressed the wife did not attend the surgery. Possibly she had less time to think about her own symptoms.

It was found that the longer the chart, i.e. the longer the time-span investigated, the easier it was to observe periods of apparent family ill health.

No. 32

	1958												1959												1960					
	1	2	3	4	5	6	7	8	9	10	11	12	1	2	3	4	5	6	7	8	9	10	11	12	1	2	3	4	5	6
Mother 41				D	I	RV RV I	H RV		F									F										I	RV RV F	
Daughter 19		F	DDR F P		F		D	D DR RV									I										F	I P	F P F	
Father 42					I P	RVP	Pr	Pr 2									F F P					I				I	FO RV RVRV RVRV			I
Son 9	D DR DR						D DR F		D	RV	Rec									I		I								

FAMILY 32

4 in household. Father, 42, baker. Mother, 41, housewife. Daughter, 19, shorthand typist. Son, 9, at school.

The three adult members of the family tend to have neurotic symptoms.

Feb.-May 1958. Daughter had various hypochondriacal symptoms. This was probably due to a mild depression.

May-Aug. 1958. Father had a mild anxiety state.

May. Mother found to have a hypochromic anaemia due to menorrhagia and also a second degree uterine prolapse. She had an hysterectomy in July 1958.

Aug. 1958. Son had a minor behaviour disorder.

May 1959. Father attended four times between the 19th and the 30th. On the first and second attendances he complained of chest pain, next he had neurodermatitis, and on the last attendance a marked anxiety state.

3 June. Mother attended with symptoms of a mild anxiety state.

D

March 1960. Husband had a tennis elbow. He attended five times for injections of hydrocortisone acetate.

March-June 1960. Daughter had a mild depression.

May. Mother injured her leg. She had a wound which took four weeks to heal.

June. Mother attended with functional symptoms.

There is one period of ill health lasting from February until August, 1958. The mother had an organic illness and it is possible that the father's mild neurotic illness was precipitated by the ill health in the family. The son had only one minor emotional disturbance and that occurred after his mother had been an inpatient in hospital.

There were only three attendances during the next eight months. In May and June 1959 there is an example of a paired entry which was probably caused by interaction. After not attending for eight months, the wife's mild neurotic symptoms coincided with the husband's illness. During the following seven months there were only three attendances for minor organic ailments. This is followed by another period of ill health and it appears as though the father's minor disability in March 1960 had precipitated the daughter's illness. This chart also shows a 'crowding' of attendances in parts and a relative paucity in others.

No. 33

	1958												1959											
	1	2	3	4	5	6	7	8	9	10	11	12	1	2	3	4	5	6	7	8	9	10	11	12
Mother 31				I F	F P	F ECT	F		P F	F F	F		F		I	FO		///// Pregnancy /////				I	I	
Celia 4		I	I	I			2					F		I I		I								
Alma 9									F	I														
Father 35										F RV RV					F	RVP								

38

FAMILY 33

4 in household. Father, 35, aircraft painter. Mother, 31, housewife. Two daughters, Alma, 9; Celia, 4.

The mother had an endogenous depression in 1957 which was treated with electropexy while an inpatient. In 1958 she was attending a psychiatric outpatient clinic.

From April 1958 until April 1959 the mother frequently attended the surgery with either hypochondriacal or overt emotional symptoms.

The children had either minor organic ailments or, on a few occasions, symptoms for which no organic cause could be found.

There were two periods each lasting about a month when the father had mild functional symptoms.

The mother's mental state had improved after she had had ECT as an outpatient. She still had hypochondriacal symptoms and was anxious at times but not depressed. She showed insight and was apologetic about needing further reassurance that she was 'really quite healthy'.

She became pregnant in March 1959. Thereafter she showed further considerable improvement and was symptom-free, rational, and optimistic. She had an uneventful pregnancy and puerperium.

If attendance for antenatal care had been entered on the chart, the mother's part would show regular entries after April 1959 because she was still under our continuous care. However, it is of greater interest for the purposes of this investigation that she was in good mental health and that she was symptom-free during this time. (She has maintained this improvement up to the time of writing.) It is conspicuous that after the mother's mental health improved there were no attendances from other members of the family. It appears as though 'the children's symptoms had been symptoms of the mother's illness' (Balint, 1957).

No. 34

	1958												1959											
	1	2	3	4	5	6	7	8	9	10	11	12	1	2	3	4	5	6	7	8	9	10	11	12
Mother 46			P	P		FO	I	RV RV	RV S	P P P	I			I				P	P			S	I	
Father 53	F	I RV RV	F	P		I				F				FO			F	I					F	I
Daughter 16								F		F														

FAMILY 34

3 in household. Father, 53, clerk. Mother, 46, housewife. Daughter, 16, shorthand typist.

Both parents attended frequently. The father had had a coronary thrombosis in 1955. Both had frequent hypochondriacal symptoms.

The daughter attended with her mother on two occasions but no organic cause was found for the daughter's symptoms.

From August until October 1958 there was a marital crisis, because the wife found out that her husband had been unfaithful to her. In October he left her to live with another woman but returned to her in February. The husband was on another general practitioner's list while he was away.

The number of attendances was twice as high in 1958 as in 1959. During the marital crisis, from August till October, the wife attended more frequently and this was also the only period in which the daughter had mild symptoms. The wife's attendances became markedly less frequent after her husband had left her. Eight months later she had the first recurrence of emotional symptoms and, according to the patient, these were due to new marital discord.

The first three families in this group and family 23 are unusual in that the 'crowding' of attendances is clearly demarcated; the rest of the group have patterns similar to the last chart. The charts of some other families whose members attended frequently showed a greater density of entries in parts but crowding was not conspicuous.

SUMMARY

While tabulating the attendances of individual patients in a general practice it was observed that the attendances were unevenly distributed. Sometimes physical illness and minor emotional disturbances of members of the same family either coincided or closely followed each other; these attendances formed pairs and clusters on the charts. The attendance charts (for two years) of 356 families were examined. Families were investigated further in which a member had attended with neurotic symptoms.

By this means sixty families were found in which some form of interaction between members of the same family may have occurred. The families were divided into four groups.

GROUP I   Those in which at least one member attended rarely; in these families it was easier to investigate pairing and clustering of attendances (twelve families).

GROUP II   Those in which attendances were more frequent, so that paired entries and clusters were less conspicuous (ten families).

GROUP III Those whose members attended frequently. An attempt was made to find attendances owing to interactions among the other consultations. Thirty-one of these families were found, the paired attendances of ten of them have been described.

GROUP IV   Those in which the attendance rate of two or more members varied together; there appeared to be periods of 'family ill health'. Seven of these families were found and the attendances of four of these families have been described.

41

CHAPTER 3

Pairs and Clusters

When the families had been selected, an attempt was made to analyse and classify the causes of pairing and clustering. In order to estimate the incidence of interactions the pairs owing to other causes must be excluded.

CAUSES OF PAIRS AND CLUSTERS

Infection and Coincidence

Both these causes are important because they are common, but neither merits discussion at this stage. Epidemics within the family were an obvious cause for clusters on the attendance charts and many paired entries were undoubtedly coincidental.

The Maturing of a Resolution

Sometimes this phenomenon can be observed in patients who do not attend frequently. One member of a family delayed attendance at the surgery until another had begun to visit. His behaviour suggested that some time previously he had decided to seek medical advice, but his resolution did not mature until the other member became ill. The next case is an example.

42

No. 35

	1958												19 59											
	1	2	3	4	5	6	7	8	9	10	11	12	1	2	3	4	5	6	7	8	9	10	11	12
Sister 60											I	RV ZH RV P												
Brother 51										I	I RV													

FAMILY 35

6 in household. Only two members of this family were our patients. Sister, 60, unmarried. Brother, 51, single, post office sorter.

The sister kept house for four brothers and another sister living in the same household. All are single. The brother had not attended for three years and the sister for five years.

11 Oct. Brother attended complaining of a 'lump'. He was found to have a direct right inguinal hernia and my partner referred him to a surgical outpatient clinic.

19 Nov. Brother re-attended complaining of low backache. The history was suggestive of a ligamentous strain but I could find no abnormality on examination.

26 Nov. Brother re-attended; by this time the ache had improved.

30 Nov. Sister seen by my partner. She complained of vague pelvic discomfort; on examination he found that she had a large ovarian cyst and he referred her to a gynaecological outpatient clinic; her name was put on the waiting list for admission.

Dec. Sister re-attended.

Jan. She had a total hysterectomy and bilateral salpingo-oophorectomy. After discharge from hospital she attended complaining that she felt tense and could not sleep.

Feb. Sister re-attended; she was feeling better and she did not come again.

Two members of the same family did not attend for five

43

and three years respectively; then both attended within a short period of time. Both had long-standing conditions. The sister's behaviour suggested that the brother's attendances had acted as a reminder to her to seek medical advice for herself.

Many of the interactions described in the previous chapter seem to have an element of this 'maturing of the resolution': 'One of these days I must do something about this pain' or 'this discomfort' appears to be a decision previously made, but not acted upon.

This is similar to the situation where one member of a family is afflicted with toothache or takes the plunge to have dental treatment. Others are then more inclined to make the long postponed appointment for dental prophylaxis. To visit the doctor is an unpleasant decision for the patient—chiefly if he does not attend frequently—and a decision that is only too readily postponed. A neighbour's illness, an aggravation of his own symptoms, a newspaper article about disease, may all influence him, as may another illness within the family, and change the resolution into a deed.

The Escort's Symptoms

The simultaneous attendance of two members of the same family both having symptoms is a frequent cause of paired entries. This situation is well known to general practitioners. Often the escort's opening remark is a phrase such as: 'While I am here', 'To save me coming again', or 'I hope you won't mind, Doctor'. (I assume that the phraseology differs with the type of practice and the part of the country.)

A count of all entries of this sort would give a false impression of morbidity, and would also interfere with the investigation of other modes of interaction. These paired entries are different from those in which the second member decides to see his doctor and puts up with the discomfort of waiting alone his turn at the surgery.

The actual reasons for attendances in the escort pair may of course vary; two examples are given below.

No. 36

	1958												1959											
	1	2	3	4	5	6	7	8	9	10	11	12	1	2	3	4	5	6	7	8	9	10	11	12
Mother 33									F RVP															
Son 7									1 RV									D DR		D				

FAMILY 36

3 in household. Father, 37, shop manager. Wife, 33, house-wife. Son, 7.

The father attends rarely. The mother and the boy had not been to the surgery for two years.

Sept. 1958. Mother and son came to the surgery. The boy had multiple infected gingival ulcers. The gum around a socket was infected following a recent tooth extraction, and I thought that the ulcers were due to a local spread of infection.

The mother complained that she frequently felt 'dizzy', had 'no energy', and was afraid of developing cancer. She had had a thyreoglossal cyst removed many years previously and she was afraid that this was a site from which cancer could develop. I found no abnormality on examination.

Sept. One week later. Both re-attended. The boy's ulcers had almost healed and the mother was more settled, perhaps partly owing to my reassurance that she was in excellent physical health and that her present symptoms were compatible with a long life.

June and Sept. 1959. Son visited at home. On both occasions he had mild upper respiratory tract infections.

The son's infected mouth appeared to be the main reason for attendance and the mother seemed to have taken the opportunity to talk about her fears. However, although this

45

is a paired entry on account of the escort's symptoms, it is possible that the mother would eventually have sought medical advice even if she had not had to accompany her son.

The next example is similar and is of common occurrence.

No. 37

	1958												1959											
	1	2	3	4	5	6	7	8	9	10	11	12	1	2	3	4	5	6	7	8	9	10	11	12
Mother 44										1														
Daughter 15										1														

FAMILY 37

4 in household. Father, 46, railway inspector. Mother, 44, housewife. Son, 21, bus conductor. Daughter, 15, schoolgirl.

No member of the family had attended for four years. *Oct.* Mother and daughter attended together. The daughter complained of a 'sore throat'; she had pharyngitis. The mother said that she had difficulty in reading; she was found to be mildly presbyopic and was referred to an optician.

This case also presents as an escort pair and again probably some maturing of a resolution has occurred. It is likely that the mother had resolved for some time to have her eyes examined; she would probably have come in any case, but her daughter's attendance induced her to come sooner.

When visiting the patients' homes, only the illness of one member was tabulated unless definite pathology was found in another person. When it happened, as it often did, that another member of the family took the opportunity to ask for advice for a minor complaint, this was noted in the visiting book, but not included on the charts.

One would expect 'escort pairs' to occur frequently because it is rational and practical for two or more members of a family to attend together. When small children are brought

46

to the surgery by a busy mother it is reasonable for her to ask for advice at the same time; a mother may act similarly if she chaperons her adolescent daughter. One member of the family going to the surgery may invite another for company or even exhort him to 'have something done about that cough of yours'. The label 'escort' therefore indicates only that the pairing occurred on the same date. It does not indicate any particular cause.

Doubtful Interaction

This group merits a separate heading for the sake of completeness, because in an attempt to analyse the incidence of interactions many 'pairs' must be allotted to this group. If there was reason to suspect that a pair was not coincidental yet there was insufficient evidence to give it another label, it was classified under this heading.

The number of 'doubtful interactions' varies in proportion to the investigator's scepticism; many of the pairs classified below might be regarded as unrelated by others. However, it was useful to assume that interaction had occurred in order to investigate them further.

Spread of Ill Health

This is a complicated group. In this group interaction had probably occurred between two members; in some way the illness of one appeared to act as a form of stress that caused ill health in the second member. The way in which this might be brought about will be discussed below.

PAIRS AND CLUSTERS IN SIXTY FAMILIES

The apparent causes of pairing and clustering in the sixty families described in Chapter 2 were examined, and the pairs and clusters were labelled according to the apparent cause. No time limit was set for regarding two attendances as paired. In order to simplify the count only two attendances in each cluster were considered and also attendances because of

47

functional and overt emotional symptoms shared the label 'neurotic illness'. The pairs and clusters in each group were further subdivided according to the diagnosis.

TABLE 1 APPARENT CAUSES OF PAIRING AND CLUSTERING IN 60 SELECTED FAMILIES

(The figures in parenthesis indicate that another label would have been equally appropriate)

	Both illnesses organic	1st illness organic 2nd illness 'neurotic'	Both illnesses 'neurotic'	Others	Total
Spread of ill health	—	23(−12)	21(−5)	4	48(−17)
Coincidence	20	—	—	8	28
Doubtful interaction	4	5	7	9	25
Escort pairs	6	8	4	—	18
Infection	15	—	—	—	15
Resolution	12	—(+12)	—(+5)	—	12(+17)
Total	57	36	32	21	146

Comment and Discussion

Because these families were chosen by the pairs and clusters on their charts, the total number of interactions is likely to be in excess of those of a random sample and the causes are also likely to be different.

Spread of ill health. Out of 146 pairs, 48 were labelled 'spread of ill health', but 17 of these 48 could have equally been classified as 'maturing of a resolution'. In these cases a mild neurotic illness appeared to have been aggravated by the illness of another member, therefore by definition these paired entries could have been given either label. After deducting the latter this leaves 31 pairs in which illness had apparently spread from one member to another healthy member, causing him to be ill.

In a few cases a healthy member developed symptoms only after great emotional strain. For example, in family No. 10, the husband complained of symptoms only when he was alone following his wife's admission to hospital for mastectomy. In other cases, it was a minor ailment that seemed to precipitate a neurotic illness in the second member. It appears that illness in a family can produce diverse effects. Sometimes a minor illness of one member produced symptoms in the second, whereas a serious illness did not seem to affect him at all. There are, therefore, additional factors which will determine whether, and how, the second member will react. Probably his state of mental health or other strains will influence his response.

Maturing of a resolution. Twelve cases were found to be due to this phenomenon. In these cases the second illness, which was an organic one, had been present before the first member's attendance. In addition there were seventeen other cases which have been discussed in the last paragraph.

Coincidence. Twenty-eight pairs were labelled thus. These were pairs of two organic illnesses not related to each other, accidents and organic illnesses, or those pairs in which an emotional illness preceded the organic one. The organic illnesses under this heading were those which have no known psychological factor in their aetiology.

In some of these pairs the second illness was due to an infection. Since this survey has been completed Meyer and Haggerty (1962) have published an investigation on susceptibility to bacterial infection. They found that various distressing events, which included illness in the family, were more frequent in the two weeks preceding streptococcal throat infections than in the two weeks following. It is therefore possible that some of the pairs in which the second illness was due to infection, and which have been labelled in this volume as coincidence, were a form of psychosomatic interaction in the family.

Doubtful interactions. Twenty-five pairs were allotted to this group and these were chiefly pairs in Groups III and IV. In four cases the second illness was psychosomatic; these were patients who had frequent episodes of neurodermatitis or asthma and therefore a recurrence was not necessarily thought to be due to interaction.

Escorts. Eighteen pairs were due to escorts; this would have been a higher number if all the services rendered had been entered in the attendance charts. (There is no case in this series where more than two members attending together had illnesses, except for upper respiratory tract infections. If we were asked to see more members, the other complaints were minor ones.)

In twelve pairs one or both members had functional or overt emotional symptoms and this high incidence is due to the selection of these families. In one-third of the escort pairs both illnesses were organic. Therefore it is likely that some of the mechanisms already described were partly responsible.

THE ROLE OF FAMILY MEMBERS

Interactions were further investigated to assess how often various members of the family took part and whether father or mother, son or daughter differed in their emotional reactions.

Each member of the 60 families was given a label according to the position in the family. The paired entries due to spread of ill health were selected and the interactions between the various members of the family were counted. Doubtful interactions and other causes of pairing were not considered.

TABLE 2 DISTRIBUTION OF ATTENDING MEMBERS IN
60 SELECTED FAMILIES

Family relationship	M	D	F	S	Fil	Mil	H	W	B	Si	Total
Number	54	58	45	37	6	5	4	4	2	2	218

TABLE 3 'SPREAD OF ILL HEALTH' IN 60 SELECTED
FAMILIES IN TWO YEARS

1st illness	2nd illness	Number of interactions
F —	M	10
S —	M	8
M —	D	7
D —	M	6
M —	F	4 (W — H 2)
M —	S	4
Sib —	Sib	4
Mil —	Dil	1 (on two occasions)
Dil —	Mil	1 (on two occasions)
F —	D	Nil
D —	F	1
F —	S	Nil
S —	F	Nil

Total 48

The code means: M = mother. F = father. D = daughter. S = son. H = husband. W = wife.
Fil = father-in-law. Mil = mother-in-law. Dil = daughter-in-law. B = brother. Si = sister.
Sib = sibling.

The 'Families' are defined on page 59.

In these families there were 218 patients who had attended
at least once. There was a larger number of 'mothers' than
'fathers'. Four couples were labelled 'husband and wife';
these were either childless or their children lived away.

Table 3 shows that interactions between mother and
children occurred twenty-five times and between mother and
father sixteen times (including twice between 'husband and
wife'). Interaction between father and children occurred only
once, the daughter's illness following the father's.

51

Discussion

In these families various members appear in unrepresentative proportions. The difference between the numbers of mothers and fathers can be partly explained by the fact that in this sample there were four widows and in five families the father was on another general practitioner's list. There is a considerably greater number of daughters than of sons. The main reason appears to be that mothers and daughters tend to chaperon each other, therefore their attendance charts show more paired entries and this probably influenced their selection for this investigation.

The largest difference was in the number of interactions occurring between mother and children on one hand and between father and children on the other. Of the latter there were only two entries labelled 'spread of ill health' and these occurred between the same pair, father and daughter, one of them being outside the time-span investigated. Minor symptoms caused by interactions between father and children seem to be relatively rare. The total number of interactions of the children with the mother do not show a sex difference although there is a considerably larger number of daughters in these families. As the ages of the children vary considerably and the numbers are too small, no conclusions can be drawn from these figures.

The wife's illness followed the husband's almost twice as often as vice versa. One reason may be that the incidence of neurotic symptoms is greater in women than in men. The word 'illness' has been used freely in the last few paragraphs. Sometimes the word denotes an attendance for one mild functional symptom the severity of which was not as important as the fact that it occurred at a particular time. It is possible therefore that the sex difference occurred because women attend surgery more readily, thus these figures do not necessarily indicate that wives are more affected by their husband's illnesses than the reverse.

FIGURE 1

NUMBER OF INTERACTIONS IN TWO YEARS IN 60 SELECTED FAMILIES

One arrow represents about 5 interactions. The arrow points to the member of the family whose symptom followed the illness of the other member.

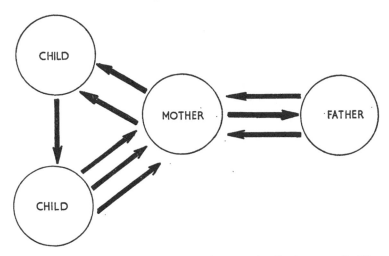

The figures can be represented graphically (*Figure 1*). The family's health seems to hinge on the well-being of the mother. Coolridge (1956) described cases in which bronchial asthma in mother and child appeared to be affected by interactions. Apley (1959) found that parental illness (usually maternal) was one of the precipitating causes of abdominal pains in children for which no organic cause could be found. Buck (1959) found a higher incidence of behaviour and psychosomatic disorders in the children of neurotic mothers but not of neurotic fathers. Rutter (1962) found that psychiatric disorders in children occurred more often with maternal mental illness than with paternal. He found, however, no difference in parental physical illness. Murstein (1960) found little difference in the emotional adjustment of mother and father in severe illness of a child.

The minor interactions described here may perhaps not

E   53

help in understanding the effects of severe or prolonged parental illness; also some of the numbers are probably biased. It appears, however, that when the father is ill, the mother who may be anxious and sad, and who may also suffer economically, may be the intermediary which distresses the children.

SUMMARY

In 60 selected families 146 paired entries and clusters were found in two years.

An attempt was made to analyse the pairs and clusters and to divide them into groups.

Those due to:
1. Identical infection in members of the same family.
2. Coincidence.
3. Paired entries due to the escort's symptoms: Chaperons or mothers attending with their children tend to ask for advice at the same time.
4. Maturing of a resolution. These were paired entries in which a patient had had an illness for some time but did not attend until another member of the family became ill. He behaved as though the other illness had acted as a reminder and as though his resolution to seek medical advice had matured.
5. Doubtful interactions.
6. Spread of ill health. These were paired entries in which the illness of one member of the family apparently caused symptoms in another member; the symptoms may have been caused by stress.

There was a considerable overlap between Groups 4 and 6.

Interaction within the Family

In forty-eight cases spread of ill health had apparently occurred.

It occurred mostly between mother and children, and only once between father and child.

CHAPTER 4

Family Attendance Rates

A general practitioner often has the impression that members of some families attend frequently whereas members of others attend hardly at all. When a member of one of the latter families comes to the surgery, he may note with surprise that they have been on his list for years, that all the case files are empty, and that he did not know of their existence. I have not investigated this group thoroughly, because these patients are somewhat inaccessible and have the good fortune to figure negatively in medical statistics. When one meets them they appear to be a sturdy lot and often boast about their good health. When they have an illness they often volunteer statements to the effect that they do not like to 'give in' or to 'bother doctors'. A mother may say of her children: 'They are quickly up and down; when they are poorly I put them to bed for a couple of days and they get better'. Exceptionally the reason for the rare attendance is ignorance or fear, but for the most part these families appear to be in vigorous health.

There are other families, in which one or more members suffers from a chronic illness. The following is an example of a family in which illness was severe and which frequently needed our help.

FAMILY 38

4 in household. Father, 57, clerk. Mother, 54, housewife. Daughter, 27, recently married. She and her husband live with her parents. They have one single son, 24, who does not live at home.

The mother has bronchial asthma, neurodermatitis, and trigeminal neuralgia. She is sensitive to salicilates and to ephedrin. The father has suffered from recurrent depressive illnesses for 26 years and has had to be admitted to mental hospitals in the past. He has a duodenal ulcer and also a severe psoriasis, which, if untreated, causes the skin to break and ulcerate. The dermatologist who treated him felt justified in prescribing oral corticosteroids, the only treatment that gave him any relief. When an exacerbation of the ulcer occurred, corticosteroids were discontinued, which caused a severe recurrence of the psoriasis. The daughter, who has a good personality, has—not surprisingly—occasional hypochondriacal symptoms.

How does the severe illness of one affect the others? Does 'spread of ill health' occur in families where illness is continuous? Hopkins (1959) described one of these families, and apparently 'transmission of illness' had occurred. Balint *et al.* (1960) have observed cases in which 'one member of the family is seriously ill and the general practitioner who is well acquainted with the other members may know that one or the other is labouring under a very heavy strain but somehow must remain healthy so that the other member may remain ill'. The families with chronic illness are usually well known to the practitioner who may have been visiting the home for many years; the reactions of the other members can be observed but are difficult to measure.

The attendance charts are usually of little value in the investigation of these families. In chronic organic illness the attendance pattern of a patient seems to be determined almost entirely by the state and the severity of the illness, though

56

sometimes other factors play a part. For instance, when starting treatment with a new drug, the doctor may ask the patient to attend more frequently and this may produce crowding of entries on the charts; conversely, when a patient is resigned that the illness cannot be cured he may call less frequently although his health has not improved.

On the assumption that attendance rates are a measure of ill health, the attendance rates of families have been investigated. The families were divided into those in which neurotic symptoms occurred and the rest. The pairs and clusters were counted in these groups and an attempt was made to assess whether interactions affected the patients' behaviour or even their health.

METHOD AND RESULTS

The first 200 families in alphabetical order were chosen for this part of the investigation and they were divided into two groups:

Group A ('*Neurotic families*'). Families in which a member attended at least once because of functional symptoms or because of an overt emotional disturbance.

Group B ('*Non-neurotic families*'). Families in which none of the above symptoms occurred during the two years of the investigation.

TABLE 4 NUMBER OF FAMILIES AND PATIENTS IN THE SAMPLE

	Group A '*neurotic families*'	*Group B* '*non-neurotic families*'	*Total*
Number of parents	126	144	270
'Husbands and wives' (childless or children live away)	40	36	76
Others (grandparents, in-laws, etc.)	16	20	36
Children[1]	135	162	297
Total number of patients	317	362	679
Number of families	97	103	200

[1] 28 of the 'children' were over 20 years of age.

57

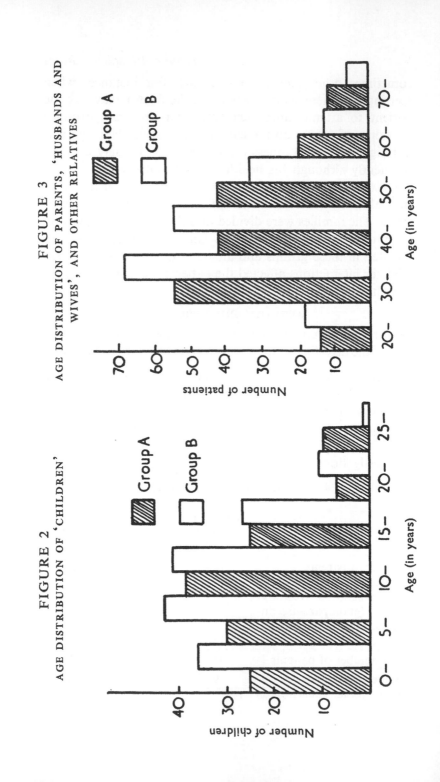

FIGURE 2

AGE DISTRIBUTION OF 'CHILDREN'

FIGURE 3

AGE DISTRIBUTION OF PARENTS, 'HUSBANDS AND WIVES', AND OTHER RELATIVES

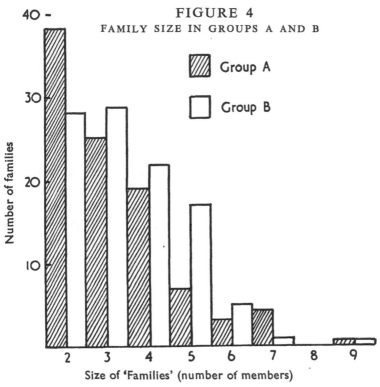

FIGURE 4

FAMILY SIZE IN GROUPS A AND B

Size of 'Families' (number of members)

There were 97 families in Group A and 103 in Group B. The number of patients was larger in the latter group. The 'families' under investigation were tabulated, but not the actual size of the family, e.g. an elderly couple whose children live in another part of the country was tabulated as a family of two members. In those families in which a member was on another general practitioner's list (7 in Group A and 11 in Group B), only the members included in this investigation were tabulated. 'Families' with two members belonged more often to Group A and larger families more often to Group B. There were fewer young children in Group A, and parents, 'husbands and wives' (childless couples or couples whose children lived away), and other relatives (grandparents, in-laws etc.) tended to be somewhat older.

Family Ill Health

Paired Attendances

Attendances because of illness were counted in each group (i.e. all attendances except those for maternity work, immunization, medical certificates, and repeat prescriptions). Revisits[1] were not considered in the counting of pairs and clusters. If more members needed consultations on a visit at home, these were not counted as pairs.

In this part of the investigation a time limit was chosen for regarding attendances as paired or clustered and this varied according to the second member's date of last attendance. The consultations of two members were counted as paired if the time interval between them was less than three weeks. If the second member had attended within the previous six months the time limit was shortened to two weeks. The same rule applied for clustering. If a third member of the same family attended within the next two or three weeks, the three attendances were counted as a cluster.

The pairs and clusters were counted in each group. Pairs due to infections and due to escorts were counted separately, as these were easily recognized. The number of the remaining pairs and clusters was compared.

The Incidence of Pairs and Clusters

There was a larger number of pairs and clusters in Group A than in Group B. The number of pairs and clusters due to infections was similar in both groups and there were more pairs due to escorts in Group A.

TABLE 5 PAIRS AND CLUSTERS IN
GROUPS A AND B IN TWO YEARS

	Pairs			Clusters			
	Escorts	Infection	Other	Escorts	Infection	Other	Total
Group A	22	17	97	—	—	23	159
Group B	10	13	21	—	4	3	51

[1] The terms 'consultation' and 'attendance' have been used freely and therefore are interchangeable; as opposed to 'revisits' which were further doctor-patient contact for the same episode of illness.

Statistical tests showed that nearly all, or perhaps all, of the increase in number of the remaining pairs in Group A was due to members of this group tending to consult considerably more often than members of Group B. There was, however, a moderately strong indication, probably significant (if an exact test were made) at the conventional 5 per cent level, of a difference between Groups A and B in families of two members. (For the statistical report see Appendix IV, pp. 105-6.)

In order to examine further the apparent causes of pairing—and this is only feasible in families whose members attend relatively rarely—families with a 'frequent attender' were excluded ('F families'). A patient was regarded as a frequent attender if he had 12 or more consultations in two years.

TABLE 6 APPARENT CAUSES OF
PAIRS AND CLUSTERS
AFTER 'F FAMILIES' HAVE BEEN EXCLUDED

	Group A	Group B
Number of families	79	98
Consultations in two years	955	570
Pairs due to:		
Infection	11	9
Escorts	19	11
'Spread of ill health'	20	2
'Resolution'	10	7
Doubtful interactions	14	2
Coincidence	41	11
Total number of pairs	115	42

There were 18 'F families' in Group A and 5 in Group B. In the remaining families there were 100 pairs and 15 clusters in Group A and 38 pairs and 4 clusters in Group B. In labelling the clusters, only the first two consultations were

61

considered. The incidence of pairs due to infection and resolution was similar in both groups. The largest difference was in the pairs labelled spread of ill health. There were only two pairs in Group B and in both cases the second consultation was due to asthma.

Attendance Rates

In order to calculate the attendance rates both groups were corrected to 100 families each.

In Group A the next three 'neurotic families' were added and in Group B the last three families were excluded. The groups were renamed A1 and B1. There were 8 families totalling 19 patients who had no attendances during the two years of the investigation. Members of these families had filled in the sociological questionnaire and it was ascertained that none of these patients had had an illness during the time of the investigation which was treated elsewhere, for example on holiday or at a casualty department. By definition these families were included in Groups B and B1.

TABLE 7 NUMBER OF ATTENDANCES IN TWO YEARS
Group A1 ('neurotic families') and Group B1 ('non-neurotic families')

	Number of families	Number of members	Consulta-tions	Revisits	Total attendances
Group A1	100	329	1,508	752	2,260
Group B1	100	353	657	505	1,162
Total	200	682	2,165	1,257	3,422

Group A1 had a somewhat smaller number of patients than Group B1 yet their total number of attendances was almost twice as high as in Group B1. The difference was greater between consultations than between revisits.

TABLE 8 ATTENDANCES OF PATIENTS WHO HAD NEUROTIC
SYMPTOMS AND THOSE OF THEIR RELATIVES IN TWO YEARS[1]

	Number of patients	Consultations	Revisits	Total attendances
Patients who had 'neurotic' symptoms	147	980	354	1,334
Relatives of the above patients	182	528	398	926
Total in Group A1	329	1,508	752	2,260

[1] Tables showing the age distribution are included in Appendix III.

TABLE 9 ATTENDANCE RATES FOR GROUPS A1 AND B1

	Group A1	Group B1	'Neurotic patients'	Relatives of 'neurotic patients'
Consultations	2·3	0·9	3·3	1·5
Revisits	1·1	0·7	1·2	1·1
Total attendances	3·4	1·6	4·5	2·5
Ratio consultations/ revisits	2·0	1·3	2·8	1·3

Group A1 was further divided into two sub-groups. First, those patients who had attended with neurotic symptoms and, second, their relatives. The attendance rate was the number of attendances per patient in one year. The patients who had neurotic symptoms had the highest attendance rates and the ratio of consultations to revisits was higher than in other patients. Their relatives had higher attendance rates than the patients in Group B1.

In Group A1 there were 147 patients who had neurotic symptoms and of these 129 were adults. In the original sample (i.e. Groups A and B) 21·5 per cent of all members and 32 per cent of adults had attended once in two years with neurotic symptoms. The ratio of adult women to men with these symptoms was somewhat less than 5:2.

63

FIGURE 5
ATTENDANCE RATE OF PATIENTS WITH NEUROTIC SYMPTOMS AND THAT OF THEIR RELATIVES

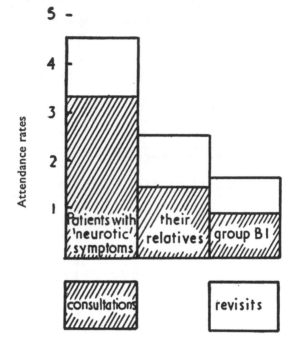

FIGURE 6
NUMBER OF PATIENTS WHO HAD CONSULTED IN TWO YEARS

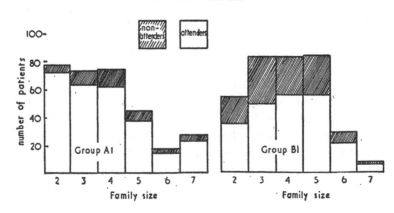

The patients who had attended were tabulated separately from those who had no attendance during the time of the survey. Group A1 had a larger proportion of patients who had attended; there were 69 families in Group A1 in which all members had attended and 5 in which only one had done so. The figures for Group B1 were 33 and 17.

In order to examine the cause of the difference in attendance rates, the attendances of patients suffering from a physical illness were counted. The illnesses were divided into acute, recurrent, and chronic. An illness was acute when it confined a previously healthy patient to bed for two weeks or more or required his admission to hospital for one week or more. A recurrent illness was a physical illness which recurred three times or more in the same year.

TABLE 10 PATIENTS WHO HAD PHYSICAL ILLNESSES
AND THEIR ATTENDANCES IN TWO YEARS

	Number of patients			
	'Neurotic patients'	*Their relatives*	*Total A1*	*B1*
Patients with chronic or recurrent physical illness	20	14	34	21
Patients with acute physical illness	7	9	16	14
Others	120	159	279	318
Total	147	182	329	353
	Attendances[1]			
Patients with chronic or recurrent physical illness	325+82	120+ 69	445+151	211+144
Patients with acute physical illness	59+ 43	12+ 26	71+ 69	22+ 32
Others	596+229	396+303	992+532	424+329
Total	980+354	528+398	1,508+752	657+505

[1] The figures represent all the attendances from whatever cause.
The first figure represents consultations and the second revisits.

65

There was a larger number of patients with physical illness in Group A1 and their attendances were partly responsible for the higher rates of the group.

TABLE 11 NUMBER OF PATIENTS WITH SOME PSYCHOSOMATIC DISORDERS IN GROUPS A1 AND B1

| | Group A1 | | | |
	Patients with neurotic symptoms	*Relatives*	*Total in Group A1*	*Group B1*
Asthma	3	2	5	4
Migraine	3	2	5	1
Peptic ulcer	1	2	3	4
Premenstrual tension	9	1	10	1

The incidence of some psychosomatic disorders was investigated. It was similar in both groups except for that of the premenstrual tension syndrome which was significantly higher in Group A1; all but one of these women also had neurotic symptoms. Migraine occurred more often in Group A1 but the difference did not reach the level of significance.

Families whose members attended frequently were selected in order to investigate further the causes of their high atten-· dance rates. Families in which the average consultation rate (excluding revisits) exceeded 2·5 for each member were labelled high attendance rate families (HARF). These families were largely in Group A1.

TABLE 12 THE INCIDENCE OF HIGH ATTENDANCE RATE FAMILIES IN GROUPS A1 AND B1

	Group A1	*Group B1*	*Total*
High attendance rate families	26	5	31
Remaining families	74	95	169
Total	100	100	200

TABLE 13 CONSULTATIONS AND REVISITS OF PATIENTS FROM
HIGH ATTENDANCE RATE FAMILIES IN TWO YEARS

	Number of families	Number of patients	Consulta- tions	Re- visits	Total visits
High attendance rate families	31	94	763	328	1,091
Remaining families	169	588	1,402	929	2,331
Total	200	682	2,165	1,257	3,422

Table 13 shows that 94 patients belonged to high attendance rate families, i.e. about one-seventh of the patients investigated. Their number of attendances was somewhat less than one-third of the total.

TABLE 14 ILLNESSES OF MEMBERS IN HIGH
ATTENDANCE RATE FAMILIES

Illnesses of members	Number of families
One member with a chronic physical illness	8
Two members with a chronic physical illness	1
One member with a psychiatric illness	8
Two members with a psychiatric illness	3
One member with mild mental ill health	4
Two members with mild mental ill health	2
Rare neurotic symptoms in one or more members	4
No neurotic symptoms and no serious physical illness	1

'Psychiatric illness' was defined as an abnormality that had interfered at least once with the patient's occupation or.

when referred to a psychiatric clinic, was diagnosed as such. 'Mild mental ill health' was an abnormality of a lesser degree.

In 8 families one member had a chronic physical illness; 3 of these belonged to Group B1. There were 30 patients in this survey who had psychiatric illness; of these 14 belonged to the high attendance rate families. Three of them were diagnosed at outpatient clinics as psychotic (2 involutional depressions and one agitated depression). Another 34 patients in these families had attended with neurotic symptoms.

In 9 families the high attendance rate was due to one member only and the others attended rarely. In 5 of these the ill member had a physical illness and in 4 a psychiatric illness. In the remaining families the attendances of two or more members contributed to the high attendance rate.

In 5 families there was no illness of importance; the high rate was largely due to minor ailments. Mild emotional symptoms were rare and they occurred in 4 of these families.

DISCUSSION

The main criticism of this part of the investigation is that it is not a random sample which has been studied, but the patients from one practice. In the first place the population was limited to a small geographical area, and in the second place patients tend to select their doctors. This selection by patients is of greater importance when investigating those conditions in which psychological factors play a part in the aetiology and is less so where physical illnesses are concerned. Therefore the incidence of illnesses in this sample may not be the same as in the total population but it is valid to compare the patients within the practice.

For the purpose of comparison the sample was divided into two groups. This grouping can be criticized on a number of counts. A patient who once in two years asks for advice about a discomfort for which no organic cause can be found cannot be diagnosed as neurotic from any but the ideal standpoint. Even less do his family, who may be in robust health, merit the description neurotic family. The term was therefore merely a convenient label, and the possibility of diagnostic errors and wrong grouping will be discussed below. If only families which had a member with a psychiatric illness had been chosen, the results would probably have been different; but research on the effect of severe mental illness on a relative is better based on a psychiatric unit if only because of the adequate number of cases available there. On the other hand, minor ill health, and the significance of minor symptoms—which are sometimes early symptoms—can be studied in general practice and an attempt was made here to use them as an indicator of strain in families.

Unfortunately, the terms used to describe minor mental ill health in general practice have to be defined. The method used here is in accordance with that of Backet, Shaw, and Evans (1953), by which an illness was defined as any disturbance in the patient's health resulting in at least one consultation. Kessel (1960) used the above method, but his term 'conspicuous psychiatric morbidity' appears to be limited to a more severe abnormality than those which were defined for the purposes of this investigation.

It could be pointed out that if the investigation had lasted long enough almost all the families could have been labelled neurotic families. Paulet (1956) found that after 6 years all but 5·5 per cent of adults underwent a physical examination for a 'neurotic disorder'. This figure seems somewhat high compared with those from this practice, but other investigations bear out his finding that the longer the time span, the larger is the proportion of patients who will have attended with symptoms of minor mental ill health. It appears therefore that if the time span investigated had been longer more families would have been in Group A; a different criterion would have been necessary to divide the sample into two roughly equal sized groups. It is also probable that if another time span had been investigated some families would have changed their groups, i.e. some which in this investigation

F   69

were placed in Group A would have been in Group B and vice versa. It seems, therefore, that this method does not differentiate between two groups of families whose characteristics are permanent except perhaps in families with chronic mental illness; it probably shows in most families only the presence or absence of neurotic symptoms at the time of the investigation.

Smaller families belonged more often to Group A. They seem to be a vulnerable group; they include childless couples, an elderly widowed parent living with a single son or daughter, etc. Although some of the figures indicating the size of the family were artificial, they suggest that mild neurotic symptoms occurred more often in smaller families and smaller households.

There are fewer patients in the 20-30 age group and this is due to the type of practice; young married couples who are childless or have only small families are not entitled to Corporation houses. Patients in Group A were somewhat older than in Group B. This age distribution appeared to be due to the somewhat higher incidence of neurotic symptoms in older women.

I have tried to use a simple method for counting pairs and clusters; in shortening the time limit for patients who had attended recently some of the pairs due to chance have probably been eliminated, since there is a large number of pairs in families which have frequent attenders. If a fixed time limit had been used, the number of pairs in Group A would have been larger.

The pairs due to escorts and infections are unlikely to be mistaken. It might have happened that two patients attended on the same day and came to different surgeries, and that these attendances bearing the same date were erroneously labelled as an escort pair. Possibly coincidental infections of two members were thought to be due to infection in the family. The first error was probably rare and the second is of minor importance for this investigation. The number of escort pairs was proportionate to the higher number of attendances, while the number of pairs due to infections was almost the same in the two groups. The number of remaining pairs and clusters was higher in Group A but contrary to expectation they were only proportionate to the larger number of attendances and to the larger number of members attending. There appeared to be a considerably larger number of pairs due to 'spread of ill health' in Group A, but since neurotic symptoms or psychosomatic illness were necessary to label a pair such, the difference in the two groups is obviously biased. A possible explanation for these findings is that spread of ill health does not exist and that all pairs are coincidental, but this would deny, *inter alia*, the occurrence of reactive depressions and anxiety states following disastrous illness in the family. Perhaps a longer time interval is necessary for the majority of these interactions to produce symptoms. It is possible that other mechanisms produce pairing in Group B because patients who attend rarely may need more inducement to visit their doctor. The examination of some of the pairs suggests that this may be so.

There was a larger number of pairs in Group A in 'families' of two members and the difference probably reached the level of significance of 5 per cent, but in view of all the factors which might influence the result this difference can be regarded only as suggestive. It is possible, owing to the strong emotional bond which exists in some of these families, that illness could have a greater effect on the remaining member than on those of larger households.

During the two years of the investigation 32 per cent of the adults attended with at least mild symptoms of mental ill health. Watts (1956) estimated that at least 5 new patients out of every 1,000 in general practice suffer from endogenous depressions each year. Apart from three psychotic depressions, some of the psychiatric symptoms recorded in this survey were probably due to mild affective psychoses, but I have tried to avoid using diagnostic labels in minor mental

71

ill health. The above percentage is not the true incidence for the practice as only adults living with relatives were considered. Had patients been included who lived alone or in lodgings (e.g. widows or widowers, divorcees, and single patients) the figure would probably have been higher. Other workers using similar criteria have found comparable figures. Pougher (1955), in a predominantly working-class practice in Leamington Spa, reviewed 500 consecutive patients for one year and found 'evidence of neurosis' in 36 per cent of adults. In a report prepared by a working party of the Council of the College of General Practitioners (1958) it was concluded that occurrence of neurotic symptoms in 30 per cent of patients was a 'generally accepted figure'. The incidence of clinical neurosis is, however, considerably lower. Fry (1954), in a middle-class practice in Kent, estimated the incidence of psychoneurosis and found 11·3 per cent and 12·4 per cent in two consecutive years. Kessel (1960), in a London working-class practice, found a one-year prevalence rate of 9 per cent of 'conspicuous psychiatric morbidity' and 5 per cent for 'other patients with abnormal personality'. Pemberton (1949) and Logan and Cushion (1958) have found lower figures. Logan found in his large survey that 6·5 per cent of patients consulted their general practitioner with mental and psychoneurotic disorders, but there were also other patients with symptoms of 'nervousness', 'fatigue', 'depression', etc. which may have been due to neurosis and which are not included in the above figure.

The ratio of women to men having attended with neurotic symptoms is similar to that found by others. Fry (1957) found that ratio about 3:1 and Logan somewhat over 2:1. Other investigations in general practice show a ratio between these two and it does not seem to depend on the diagnostic criteria used.

The families were divided into Groups A and B according to the symbols on the attendance charts and an apparent fault of this method is that an error of diagnosis on one occasion could have placed a family in the wrong group. Some attendances for minor ailments may have been wrongly labelled, so that some entries which read 'gastritis' or 'lumbago' may have been in fact functional symptoms, and the reverse may also have occurred. Also the more often a patient attended the more was he exposed to the risk of having a symptom labelled as functional or having a normal apprehension mistaken for a symptom of neurosis, and an error of this sort could have markedly altered the attendance rate for each group. There was therefore a bias for individual patients who attended frequently (and this includes the physically ill) to acquire the label neurotic. But there were also other causes for the association of physical illness and neurotic symptoms. In some patients there was a double pathology of physical and mental illness; in a few others—for example in epileptic patients—the psychological symptoms were a direct consequence of the disease. Some patients suffering from chronic physical illness had also mild hypochondriacal symptoms, and mild neurotic symptoms occurred sometimes during convalescence. Therefore many attendances because of physical illness had contributed to the high rate of the 'neurotic' patients. However, high attendance rates for neurotic patients have also been found by others and so has the association between physical and neurotic illness (Downes and Simon 1953). Finally, the higher rate in Group A1 was partly determined by that of the relatives who themselves had no neurotic symptoms. There was also a bias for whole families with high attendance rates—whatever the cause—to acquire the label neurotic family, but there were only a few families in which one diagnostic error could have resulted in wrong grouping. In many families there was no doubt which was the appropriate group; in some a patient had a conspicuous neurotic illness, in others a patient attended repeatedly with functional symptoms or more members of the same family had these symptoms.

Fry (1954) found the average attendance rate in a year for

psychoneurotic patients to be 6 and for the rest of the practice 3·5. These rates are higher and the ratio lower than in the present investigation but the figures are not comparable because of the different method used.

The 'relatives of the neurotics' had a higher attendance rate than the patients in Group B1 and the reasons seem to be the following: the latter group included 19 patients who belonged to families whose members had not attended during the two years and this slightly lowered the rate for the group. In some cases a patient who had no neurotic symptoms himself was gravely ill, therefore needed frequent consultations, and the husband or wife attended with symptoms of anxiety or depression that seemed to be a direct consequence of the severe strain. Therefore in such cases a severely ill patient by definition acquired the label 'relative of a neurotic'. An examination of the figures showed that mothers with small children in Group A1 brought them somewhat more often to the surgery than mothers in Group B1 and also more adult relatives had attended in the former group.

Logan found that 67 per cent of all the patients in his survey consulted their doctor at least once in one year, with wide variation between individual practices. (The percentage of patients attending was somewhat lower in this survey when calculated for one year.) He also found that the 'rate of patients consulting' was highest in the 0-15 age range. In Group B1 there is a larger number of children, yet the proportion of patients consulting was lower. These findings can only partly be explained on the higher incidence of physical illness in Group A1. There were some families in which the high attendance rate was due to minor complaints and apparently to a habit of attending the surgery and these families were more often in Group A1.

The incidence of the premenstrual tension syndrome was significantly higher in Group A1 but within the group it was almost entirely limited to women who had neurotic symptoms. Rees (1953) found a larger incidence of the premenstrual tension syndrome in women suffering from a psychiatric illness than in normal women. An investigation in this practice showed that more women with premenstrual tension had neurotic symptoms than a matched control group (Kellner, 1962). Therefore the association between neurosis and this syndrome determined the incidence in Group A.

The smaller proportion of revisits in patients who had neurotic symptoms seems to be contrary to everyday experience. Paulet (1956) found that treated neurotics were slower to recover after a physical illness than other patients. The revisit rate is partly determined by the general practitioner; he chooses how often to revisit a patient at home and also asks the patient to re-attend a certain number of times following the illness. It was sometimes difficult to choose the correct label. A later attendance with a new hypochondriacal symptom may have been labelled as a consultation in one patient, while a persisting bronchitis could have been labelled as a revisit in another. Finally, this method tends to show a larger proportion of revisits in severe acute illness and a smaller one in minor ailments and recurrent or chronic illness, and the 'neurotic' patients often suffered from the latter group of illnesses.

Owing to the definition of 'high attendance rate families', almost one-third of the families acquired the label because of one member, but had a different criterion been used— e.g. that at least two members should exceed the average yearly minimum—the distribution of these families in Groups A1 and B1 would have remained similar. Although the distribution depended on the method used, the findings showed an association between mental illness in the family and high attendance rates. Almost half of the patients with psychiatric illness belonged to the high attendance rate families and it seemed that psychiatric illness more often than physical illness occurred together with high attendance rates of other members.

CHAPTER 5

A Summing-Up

In this section an attempt is made to summarize some effects of illness in the family. The effects of genetic, social, and economic factors and 'assortative mating' (Slater and Wood-side, 1951) must contribute to a varying extent to the findings, but they were outside the scope of this work and are not dealt with here.

This volume has considered all the illnesses in a general practice and therefore many of them are minor ailments. The patient's attendance at the surgery or a request for a visit at home was regarded as the unit of illness. The attendance rates are objective findings but they are not always a reflection of morbidity; they depend partly on the habit of attending the surgery and this varies from one family to another. There is an association between neurosis and frequent attendances. Fry (1954) found that in general practice patients suffering from psychoneurosis had a high attendance rate. In this survey, their relatives attended more frequently than patients from other families. Physical illness was more common in families from which a member had attended with neurotic symptoms. It is likely that interactions were partly responsible for the last two findings.

Some interactions are well known to the general practitioner; following a tragedy in the family he may be called upon to console or treat a close relative. Others, less conspicuous but often recognized by him, are some of those attendances in which the presenting symptoms appear to be the least important. Pasmore (1959) mentions the case of a woman who complained of a trivial soreness of her forefinger to spend the rest of the time talking about the shortcomings of her husband. Interactions can be noticed by examining family attendance charts which show that the illness of one member apparently caused symptoms in another. Spread of ill health can present in several ways. Most often a patient's mild neurosis is aggravated by illness in the family. Sometimes a healthy person may have reactive symptoms if there is severe illness in the family; or a patient may have been living under some strain and the minor illness of a relative appears to have been the last straw. In some patients the symptoms are a hypochondriacal copy of another member's illness. A neighbour's or a friend's illness, or a television programme about disease, may produce a similar effect. Apley (1958), investigating children with recurrent pains for which no organic cause could be demonstrated, found that often a similar pattern of symptoms existed in the family. There are many clinical observations in the literature in which the course of a psychosomatic illness was apparently influenced by events in the family. Recently Meyer and Haggerty (1962) have shown that emotional strains in the family may predispose to streptococcal infections.

Paired attendances due to spread of ill health are rare and are only a small fraction of all the attendances in general practice; these pairs are therefore unlikely to affect the attendance rates. Most interactions which produce symptoms or affect the attendance rates probably take a longer time to do so.

The effect of illness in the family seems to depend on its severity, duration, and type, on the emotional bond between the patient and the relative, and on the susceptibility of the latter. This can be illustrated by observation of children. Bowlby (1952) regards chronic illness in a parent, especially the mother, as one of the causes of deprivation in children. Rutter (1962) found that parental physical illness was associated with psychiatric disorders in children only if the illness was chronic or recurrent. The children were more affected by parental psychiatric illness. Cowie (1961), in a study of children of psychotic parents, found that the neurotic disturbance of the children varied with the age of the child and with the type of parental illness. Parental neurosis affecting the child has been frequently described; the child may suffer from effects of marital discord or from the insecure or frightening atmosphere created by the illness. Many findings point to the maternal illness as being more damaging, chiefly in young children; in older children paternal illness seems to play an increasing part. The minor interactions in this survey suggest that in paternal illness a distressed mother may be the intermediary who affects the children. Mothers appeared to be more affected by the illness of children than did fathers.

The effect of illness on a close adult relative seems to depend largely on his personality and on his state of mental health at the time, but the other factors enumerated above also play some part. Post and Wardle (1962) have recently reviewed the literature on neurosis and psychosis in the family. There is evidence to suggest that illness in the family can have a marked effect on adults. Penrose (1944) and Gregory (1959) investigated husbands and wives who had both been admitted to mental hospitals; they concluded that the excess of mental illness in spouses may have been partly due to the effect of the first illness. Buck (1962) similarly found an excess of neuroses in both spouses in the later years of marriage but not in the early years nor before the marriage took place. Downes and Simon (1953) found a higher incidence of physical illness and psychosomatic illness in the families of psychoneurotics than in other families. One of the causes of this association may be the strain of living with a physically ill relative.

It seems that illness in the family, chiefly severe and prolonged illness, can make the relatives unhappy or afraid or can produce a preoccupation with disease. This may induce them to consult their general practitioner more often; it may sometimes precipitate neurotic symptoms or psychosomatic disorders, and perhaps predispose to physical illness.

There are probably some attendances in general practice when the doctor is unaware that the complaint is not the only reason for coming to the surgery. The complaint may be easily treated and easily cured and the hidden stress may be a minor one. If it was the outcome of an interaction it may have been short-lived and unimportant. I hope that by tabulating the family attendances some of these interactions have been revealed.

SUMMARY[1]

The attendance rates of families in a general practice have been investigated. The first two hundred families were chosen for this part of the investigation, and these were divided into two groups.

Group A. In which a member had at least one consultation in two years because of functional symptoms or an overt emotional disturbance.
Group B. In which none of the above symptoms occurred.

The families tended to be smaller and the average age was somewhat higher in Group A.

A time limit was chosen for regarding the consultations of two members of the same family as paired. Those due to escorts and infections are easily identified and were excluded. The number of remaining pairs was considerably higher in

[1] Summaries of Chapters 2 and 3 appear on pp. 41 and 54.

Group A, but this was apparently only due to the larger number of consultations. There was a suggestive increase in the number of pairs in Group A in 'families' of two members.

In order to calculate the attendance rates, these groups were corrected to make two groups comprising 100 families each: Group A1 and Group B1. The attendance rate of patients in Group A1 was twice as high as that of patients in Group B1. Patients who had neurotic symptoms had the highest attendance rate. The rate of their relatives was lower but still higher than that of patients in Group B1. The proportion of patients who had attended was higher in Group A1; there was a higher incidence of physical illness in Group A1 which also contributed to the high rate of the group.

The incidence of the premenstrual tension syndrome was significantly higher in Group A1 but this was almost entirely limited to women who had neurotic symptoms. The difference in the number of patients suffering from migraine was only suggestive.

High attendance rate families were defined and investigated. The incidence of psychiatric illness was considerably higher in these families than in the others.

The effects of interactions following illness in the family have been discussed.

APPENDIX I

Attendance Charts

A description now follows of the method used in compiling the attendance charts and in choosing the symbols for the consultations.

TABLE 15 THE CODE USED IN THE ATTENDANCE CHARTS IN CHAPTERS 1 AND 2

CO = Chronic organic illness	Consultation at the surgery because of a chronic organic illness.
CP = Chronic psychiatric illness	Consultation at the surgery because of a chronic neurotic or psychotic illness.
D = Domiciliary visit	Consultation at home because of an organic illness.
DP = Domiciliary visit, psychiatric	Consultation at home because of neurotic or psychotic symptoms.
ECT	Electro-convulsive therapy as an outpatient.
F = Functional symptoms	Consultation at the surgery because of somatic symptoms without an apparent organic cause.
FO = Functional overlay	Consultation at the surgery because of an organic illness and also functional or emotional symptoms.

81

H = Hospital	Stay in a hospital.
I = Illness	Consultation at the surgery because of an organic illness.
P = Psychiatric illness	Consultation at the surgery because of neurotic or psychotic symptoms.
Pr = Prescription	Attendance at the surgery for a repeat prescription.
Rec = Recurrent illness	Consultation at the surgery for an organic illness which was not a chronic illness but tended to recur in the same patient.
RV = Revisit	Revisit at the surgery because of an organic illness.
RVP = Revisit, psychiatric	Revisit at the surgery because of a neurotic or psychotic illness or because of persistent functional symptoms.
? = ?Functional	Doubtful diagnosis: It was not known whether there was an organic cause for the symptom or not.

On a few occasions other symbols were used, e.g. combinations like DCO—(Domiciliary visit—chronic organic illness).

These symbols were used in the original protocol, and some are of lesser significance in the present investigation.

Sometimes it was difficult to decide which label to use—whether, for example, to regard frequent bronchitis or otitis media as a recurrent illness or as a chronic illness. As a general rule an illness was regarded as recurrent if the patient was free of symptoms and had no abnormal signs or disabilities between the periods of illness.

The distinction between 'functional' symptoms on one hand and 'psychiatric illness' on the other is of some value, because a functional symptom can sometimes simulate other symptoms in the family. The distinction between the two was not intended as a measure of severity of the condition.

Further services during the same episode of illness were labelled revisits. The following method was used for counting 'consultations' and 'revisits', but the distinction between the two was sometimes arbitrary. A patient who had pneumonia and required eight visits would have a count of 1 consultation + 7 revisits. A bronchitic patient who had five attacks of bronchitis and who on each occasion had to re-attend once would have a count of 5 consultations + 5 revisits. Therefore a spontaneous attendance by the patient (even in cases of chronic or recurrent illness) was given a different label from further doctor-patient contacts. The aspect of the patient's behaviour investigated was his decision to seek advice from his general practitioner; revisits may be partly or entirely initiated by the latter.

Attendances for a repeat prescription only were not tabulated. Although it is an item of service, the stock of medicine in the home may be decisive and the date of attendance need not have any bearing on the illness. Also families who had a member with a chronic illness would have disproportionately high attendance rates. For the purpose of illustration these attendances were sometimes recorded on the chart but were not counted.

Illnesses in which the patient had abnormal signs were labelled organic, for example, asthma or neurodermatitis, even if an apparent emotional stress precipitated the condition, but when I considered that there was a psychological factor in the aetiology I commented on it in the text.

Formal sessions of minor psychotherapy by appointment were not included in the charts. These could have been labelled revisits, but this would have given a wrong impression of the severity and duration of the illness. Psychotherapy was sometimes continued when the patient would otherwise have ceased to attend. More severe cases of neurotic illness were referred to psychiatric outpatient clinics, and once they started to attend there the attendances at the surgery became less frequent.

Appendix I

Attendances for maternity care were not recorded in the illness charts nor the complications of pregnancy or puer-perium. If antenatal and postnatal care had been included the attendance rate for young women would have been disproportionately high. Complicating illnesses which were not due to the pregnancy were recorded as attendances.

Attendances of Families in Groups III and IV

GROUP III. FREQUENT ATTENDERS

The paired and clustered attendances of ten families in Group III are given. The features of this group have been described in Chapter 2 (p. 35).

FAMILY 21

5 in household. Father, 48, nurseryman. Mother, 48, factory worker. Three children, John, 14; Peter, 8; Mary, 6.

Number of attendances in the course of the two years (excluding revisits): Mother 9, Mary 5, Peter 4, John 2, father nil.

27 Jan. 1958. Mother came with John to surgery. She told me that he had complained of pain in his neck. I could find no abnormality on examination.

30 Jan. Both re-attended. The child's neck was better, but the mother told me that she had a low backache. This appeared to be due to a mild sacroiliac strain. She had other symptoms also, which appeared to be functional.

30 Sept. 1958. Mother came with Mary and Peter to the surgery. She told me that both children had been wetting the bed at night. She also said that Mary was 'peevish'.

On examination Mary appeared well but Peter had developed a habit spasm.

7 Oct. 1959. Mother visited at home. She complained of 'stomach pains', which she described by pointing to her epigastrium. The pain was vague, it was not related to food, and there were no aggravating or relieving factors. She had eaten breakfast and had had a normal bowel action. On examination her pulse and temperature were normal. The abdomen was soft and there was no tenderness.

10 Oct. Mother came with Peter to surgery. She told me that he was 'drinking all the time'. On examination he looked well. I could not find anything abnormal. His urine did not contain sugar and the specific gravity was 1018. I reassured the mother and told her to bring the boy again if he did not improve.

12 and 20 Oct. Mother attended alone. On both occasions she had symptoms which appeared to be functional. Peter has had no recurrence of his symptoms.

The cause of the first paired entry in January is doubtful. In September both children had a minor emotional disturbance at the same time. In October Peter's 'excessive drinking' coincided with the mother's minor neurotic illness. All the other attendances of the children were due to organic illnesses.

FAMILY 22

A 'family' of four. Father, 52, coal merchant. Mother, 54, housewife. Son, 29, clerk. Daughter-in-law, 29, housewife.

Number of attendances: Mother 7, daughter-in-law 5, son 4, father 1. The two generations live in separate households but there are close family ties.

10 Sept. Daughter-in-law attended surgery and complained of epigastric pain three hours after meals, relieved by food, milk, and alkalies. The pain had woken her in the early morning hours on two occasions. I did not investigate her fully; I assumed that it was an acute erosion because it was the first time that she had had this sort of pain, and I treated her with milk, diet, and alkalies. The pain lasted for five days and she re-attended on two more occasions. I discharged her after giving routine advice about frequent meals, avoidance of salicylates, etc.

11 Sept. Mother came to surgery and complained of having lost weight. I detected no abnormality on examination and the results of investigations were within normal limits.

30 Sept. Mother re-attended and I asked her to come again if she lost more weight.

2 April 1959. Daughter-in-law attended surgery and again complained of epigastric discomfort after meals. This was relieved after a few days' treatment.

3 April. Mother attended and complained that she had lost weight. She also had functional symptoms.

24 April. Mother re-attended. This time her weight was stationary.

On two occasions the mother-in-law attended one day after her daughter-in-law had done so and complained of loss of weight. Since this investigation started and until the time of writing (March 1961) these were the only two occasions on which she complained of losing weight.

FAMILY 23
6 in household. Father, 32, semi-skilled factory worker. Mother, 29, housewife. Two children, Julia, 5; Michael, 2. The house belongs to the paternal grandfather and grandmother, 59 and 57, who live in the same household.

The mother is asthmatic and the son has recurrent eczema. Number of attendances: Michael 10, mother 7, grandmother 7, Julia 4, father 2, grandfather 1.

4 April 1958. Mother brought Julia to surgery with otitis media.

11 April. Mother brought Michael, who had eczema.

12 April. Grandmother attended, with eczema on both hands and forearms.

10 Oct. Mother came to surgery with Michael, and complained that he was restless at night. I could find nothing abnormal on examination.

14 Oct. Grandmother attended; she complained of her skin being 'itchy' and also of suffering from headaches. I could not find abnormal signs.

18 Oct. Mother attended, with asthma.

16 Jan. 1959. Mother came to surgery with Michael, who had a recurrence of eczema.

17 Jan. Father attended complaining that his shoulder was painful. There had been no history of injury or unaccustomed physical activity. I found no abnormal signs on examination.

Three members of this household attend frequently but definite clustering had occurred. One-third of the total attendances are crowded into the three separate weeks described above. Between March 1958 and January 1959 there were twenty-six attendances excluding revisits, whereas during the next eleven months there was only one.

FAMILY 24

2 in household. Mother, 59, shop-assistant, widow. Son, 19, apprentice fitter.

The mother attended six times, the son three times, in two years. The son had registered with us when the survey started. He had not been seen by his previous general practitioner for over two years.

4 April 1958. Mother attended, with herpes zoster.

15 April. I saw the son for the first time. He complained of abdominal pain; I found nothing abnormal on examination.

12 July. Mother attended surgery and complained of a painful right knee following a fall. On examination I could find only a slight patellar tenderness.

Later the same day the son came to the surgery. He told

me that he had been losing weight for the last month. I could find no cause for this and all investigations were negative.

Dec. 1959. Son attended with bronchitis. This was his only other attendance.

The son's two attendances that had no apparent organic cause closely followed his mother's illnesses.

FAMILY 25
2 in household. Husband, 58, publican. Wife, 51, housewife; works part-time in husband's public-house. They have one son who does not live with them.

Number of attendances: Wife 7, husband 3.

Aug. 1958. Wife attended surgery and complained that she felt depressed.

Sept. Wife came with husband. She told me that she felt 'somewhat better' than at her last attendance. The husband complained of 'palpitations'. He explained that he was at times aware of his heart-beat but that he had never noticed a change in rate. I could find nothing abnormal.

Jan. 1959. Husband and wife attended together. The husband had a mild bronchitis, and the wife complained of a sore tongue. The tongue appeared to be normal on inspection.

Aug. 1959. Husband and wife again attended together. The wife had a variety of symptoms which proved to be functional. The husband told me that he had 'palpitations'. Again, the findings were not suggestive of an organic illness.

The husband had bronchitis on one occasion. On the two other attendances he complained of functional symptoms. On all three occasions, except when he came for repeat prescriptions for sedatives, he came with his wife, who had mild neurotic symptoms.

FAMILY 26

Husband, 61, foreman. Wife, 61, housewife. They have one married daughter, 38, housewife, who lives in a separate household. Three granddaughters, Carol, 19, usherette; Helen, 14, Mary 7, schoolchildren. They have one son who lives in another city.

There are close ties between the 'wife' and her daughter. Attendances in two years: Wife 9, husband 4, daughter 4, Carol 2, Helen and Mary did not attend.

17 Feb. 1958. Husband seen at home. He complained of severe retrosternal pain and was restless and agitated. I found no abnormal signs but had him admitted to a hospital. After investigations which excluded a coronary thrombosis his barium meal showed a hiatus hernia. He was discharged on 15 March.

17 March. Wife attended complaining of pain in both temples. I found nothing abnormal.

April 1959. Daughter attended, complaining that her 'nerves were bad', and also that her husband intended to leave her.

12 June, 1959. Wife attended, complaining that she felt depressed and could not sleep. She also told me that her daughter was planning separation from her husband.

13 June. Husband came to surgery. He had been attending weekly for National Insurance certificates. Two months previously he had had an exploratory arthrotomy of his right knee because of a suspected torn semilunar cartilage but no lesion was found. This time he had come for his final certificate. He told me that for the past few days he had had severe bouts of uncontrollable sneezing. He had never had hay fever, or any similar symptoms before. On examination the nasal mucosa looked grey and swollen, and had the appearance of an allergic rhinitis.

23 June. Daughter came to surgery with Carol. The daughter told me that Carol had 'nightmares' and when she tried to wake her she was 'struggling and fighting'. The girl had also fainted on one occasion. I found nothing abnormal.

Three attendances in June form a cluster. It is doubtful whether the husband's only episode of 'allergic rhinitis' was due to stress, but his daughter's marital discord resulted in overt emotional disturbance in herself, in his wife, and was perhaps responsible for the granddaughter's symptoms.

FAMILY 27

5 in household. Father, 49, joiner foreman. Mother, 42, housewife. Three daughters, Olive, 18, shorthand typist; Patricia, 17, shop-assistant; Janette, 13, schoolgirl.

Number of attendances in two years: Mother 5, father 3, Olive 3, Janette 2, Patricia 1.

27 Oct. 1958. Mother came to surgery with Janette, who had pain in the region of the left temporomandibular joint. There were no abnormal signs. The mother complained of lower back pain and of being 'all nerves'. I found that the pain was in the region of the coccyx, which was tender on examination.

29 Jan. 1959. Olive attended with acrocyanosis.

2 Feb. Mother attended complaining of cough. On further inspection it was found that she had no true cough, but she was tense and repeatedly cleared her throat. Her attitude was resentful. I found no abnormal signs.

The only two occasions on which the mother had symptoms of a minor emotional disturbance coincided with ailments of other members of the family.

FAMILY 28

4 in household. Father, 41, labourer. Mother, 42, housewife. Daughter, 19, mentally subnormal, helps mother with house-work. Son, 9, schoolboy. One son, 24, lives in another city.

The mother is hypertensive. Number of attendances: Mother 11, daughter 7, father 6, son 3.

6 June 1958. Mother came to surgery with symptoms of

91

an anxiety state. She told me that they had been evicted
from the house in which they lived and were unable to find
alternative accommodation that they could afford. The
parents were planning to live in a furnished room and the
children were to be taken into the care of the Local
Authority.

7 June. Daughter came to surgery. She told me that she
had fallen three times; she did not remember what had happened but she had found herself on the ground. No one
had seen her fall but she had bruises on her knees and hands.
I found no abnormal signs. She had not bitten her tongue
or been incontinent. She re-attended three times. I thought
at the time that she had petit mal, but before I referred her
for investigation she told me that the falling attacks had
stopped.

9 Sept.-22 Oct. Father had been attending with neurodermatitis.

16 Oct. Mother attended with cellulitis of her left leg.

25 Oct. Daughter attended, and told me that her 'wrist
kept swelling up'. The wrist looked normal and I told her
to come again if the swelling recurred.

The daughter had symptoms without an apparent organic
cause on only about two occasions, in June at the time of
her mother's anxiety state and in October when her parents
had minor ailments.

FAMILY 29

*3 in household. Husband, 32, motor mechanic. Wife, 29,
housewife. Son, 7.*

The father has hay fever and asthma. Number of attendances: Father 9, son 7, mother 6.

While the husband was in hospital for excision of a
pilonidal sinus the wife came to the surgery and complained of pain in the chest. The description of the pain was
vague, it was not related to exertion, and there were no

relieving or aggravating factors. Examination proved to be negative.

On one previous occasion the wife had a mild post-influenzal depression. Apart from this episode, the only time the wife had functional symptoms was when her husband was in hospital.

FAMILY 30
4 in household. Father, 29, fitter. Mother, 31, housewife. Two sons, Peter, 7; Victor, under 1 year.
Number of attendances: Mother 8, Peter 6, father 2, Victor 2.
Jan. 1959. Mother came to the surgery with baby. The child had a mild bronchitis and the mother complained that she had a sore throat. I could not detect any abnormality on examination.
June 1959. Mother attended with elder son who had a mild upper respiratory tract infection. The mother complained that she felt 'run down'.
Dec. 1959. Mother and elder son came together. She told me that she was afraid to leave the house and also complained that Peter had started to wet the bed.

The mother had had a mild puerperal depression in November. Apart from this she complained of functional symptoms only at the time when her children were ailing. In December the mother's mild agoraphobia and the child's bed-wetting coincided.

GROUP IV. THE UNEVEN PATTERN

This part contained details about attendances of families in Group IV. The attendance charts, summaries, and comments were presented in Chapter 2 (pp. 36-41).

FAMILY 31
5 Feb. Husband attended with cellulitis of his right index

finger. His wife came with him, complaining that she 'lost her voice occasionally'. While speaking to me her voice was normal and I found no abnormality on examination.

20 Feb. Wife attended and complained of pain in her chest, not related to exertion and not suggestive of an organic lesion. No abnormalities were discovered.

6 March. Husband attended with an abscess on his index finger.

20 March. Wife attended, complaining again of vague chest pains for which I could find no organic cause.

27 March. Wife re-attended, and told me the pain was 'better'.

9 April. Husband attended with herpes labialis.

12 April. Wife attended with a recurrence of a 'bolus hystericus'.

2 May. Wife attended, and said that she was going deaf. There was no abnormality in the external auditory meatus, the drums looked normal, and there was no objective impairment of hearing.

9 May. Husband attended and told me that he had a lump on his hand. He pointed to his capitate bone.

3 July. Husband attended complaining that he had difficulty in reading. He was found to be presbyopic and I referred him to an optician.

1 Sept. Wife attended with a recurrence of the bolus hystericus.

2 Sept. Husband seen at home. He was in bed, complained of severe pain in the lower lumbar region, and slight attempts at movement seemed to cause distressing attacks of pain. The lumbar spine was flexed and my attempts to examine him aggravated the pain. (He has severe osteo-arthritis of the lumbar spine and on a previous occasion had had a L4-L5 inter-vertebral disc protrusion.) I treated him with bed rest on boards for ten days and mobilized him gradually. He was able to return to work wearing his lumbar support at the beginning of October.

11 Nov. Wife attended and told me that she was 'jumpy' and could not relax.

29 Nov. Wife attended complaining of 'a feeling of tightness around the neck'. I found no abnormal signs.

10 Jan. Husband attended surgery with a head cold and complained of pain over his right maxillary sinus. There was no local tenderness and the sinus was translucent.

17 Jan. Husband seen at home. He had a recurrence of the backache, the pain radiating to the back of his right leg, and showed signs of a disc protrusion. The treatment was similar to that which he had had in September. It was almost two months before he was able to return to work.

8 Feb. Wife attended with a recurrence of the bolus hystericus.

23 Feb. Wife re-attended complaining of a painful back; I found no abnormal signs but was uncertain whether the pain was due to a muscular or ligamentous strain or whether it was functional.

FAMILY 32

Jan. 1958. Son had measles followed by mild bronchitis.

5 Feb. Daughter attended. She complained of vague pains in her joints. There were no abnormal signs.

3 March. Daughter seen at home. She had a mild upper respiratory tract infection.

12 March. Daughter attended complaining of a pain in the region of the right iliac fossa when walking. She also mentioned a suprapubic pain which she had had four days previously. I found nothing on examination.

19 March. Daughter re-attended and told me that she was depressed.

25 April. Mother seen at home. She had a minor inversion injury of the left ankle, having slipped and fallen the previous day.

1 May. Mother attended surgery. The ankle was less

painful, but she complained of feeling 'poorly' after a recent tooth extraction, that the 'periods were heavy' and that she was constipated. Further questioning elicited that she was suffering from menorrhagia. Her haemoglobin was 52 per cent. I treated her with oral iron and asked her to re-attend.

14 May. Daughter attended with lower backache. I found no abnormal signs.

15 May. Father attended. He complained of an 'upset stomach' and vomiting. No abnormalities were found.

26 May. Father re-attended, and complained that he was feeling 'fighting mad'. On questioning, he did not admit to any worries, nor could he give a reason for this sensation.

3 June. Mother re-attended. Vaginal examination showed that she had a second degree uterine prolapse. When her haemoglobin level had returned to normal, I referred her to a gynaecological outpatient clinic.

11 June. Father re-attended; he was now feeling less tense.

1 July. Daughter seen at home. She had a mild upper respiratory tract infection.

On 5 July the mother was admitted to hospital for an hysterectomy. She was discharged on 19 July, and re-attended on the 23rd.

10 July. Father attended, asking for a repeat prescription for sedatives.

1 Aug. Boy seen at home; he had mumps.

10 Aug. Daughter developed mumps. Both children re-visited at home.

21 Aug. Mother brought son to surgery. She told me that he was restless and that he kept 'picking his skin and picking the plaster off the wall'.

28 Aug. Father attended; he complained that he had an 'upset stomach' and 'could not sleep'.

22 Oct. Mother attended complaining that she 'felt sick immediately after meals' and also of feeling 'light-headed'. I found nothing abnormal.

Nov. Boy seen at home with mild bronchitis, which recurred in Jan. 1959.

19 May 1959. Husband attended surgery. He complained of a circumscribed chest pain strongly suggestive of being functional in origin.

23 May. Husband re-attended, still complaining of chest pain.

29 May. Husband came again with neurodermatitis.

30 May. Husband re-attended with typical symptoms and signs of an anxiety state.

3 June. Wife attended. She complained of multiple joint pains, diarrhoea when she 'got worried', and sleeplessness.

29 June. Daughter attended. She complained of a lower back pain; I detected no abnormality on examination, but the description of the pain was suggestive of a ligamentous or muscular strain.

Sept. Son had mild gastroenteritis.

Dec. Son and father had upper respiratory tract infections.

Feb. 1960. Husband attended. He had a left tennis elbow. He attended five times in March for injections of hydrocortisone acetate into the extensor origin.

23 March. Daughter attended complaining of neckache for which I could find no organic cause.

29 April. Daughter re-attended complaining of diarrhoea and vomiting.

30 April. Daughter re-attended, told me that she was 'crying without reason' and depressed.

4 May. Daughter came again and complained of pain in both iliac fossae. I found no abnormality. (On each occasion I reassured her that her symptoms were not due to an organic illness and were compatible with excellent physical health.)

8 May. Daughter re-attended and complained of a 'bad taste in the mouth'.

9 May. Daughter came again, reporting that she felt depressed.

14 May. Mother attended complaining of a sore throat, but I could find no abnormal signs.

30 May. Mother re-attended with an infected wound on her right leg.

June. Mother re-attended twice.

23 June. Husband came to surgery. He had a lower back-ache which appeared to be due to a muscular strain.

30 June. Mother attended, complaining of 'tension in the stomach'. I discovered no abnormal signs.

FAMILY 33

Feb. 1958. Celia had bronchitis.

March. Mother brought Celia to surgery with a mild pharyngitis.

9 April. Mother attended complaining that her periods were 'heavy'. Further history showed that there was probably no excessive loss of blood. I found no abnormality on examination.

21 April. Mother re-attended and complained of 'pains in the head'. No abnormality was found.

27 April. Mother brought Celia to surgery and told me that the child had cried and complained of pain during defaecation. On examination she was found to have a small tear of the anal mucosa.

2 May. Mother re-attended. She complained again of 'pains in the head', for which I found no organic cause.

28 May. Mother came to surgery and told me that she felt depressed.

27 June. Mother complained of palpitations and pain in the chest. I discovered no abnormal signs.

2 July. She complained of feeling depressed and of having lost weight.

9 July. Mother brought Celia to the surgery and told me that the child had a sore throat and that she was 'off her food'. The throat looked normal and I could find no abnormality on examination.

In the latter half of July and during August the mother had electropexy as an outpatient.

2 Sept. Mother came to the surgery, complaining of feeling 'jittery'.

19 Sept. Mother re-attended, and complained of feeling tired.

6 Oct. Mother came with Alma and told me that the child was 'deaf'. I could find no abnormality and there was no objective impairment of hearing.

10 Oct. Father attended, and complained of low backache. The ache was not localized, the description was vague, and I found no abnormality. He re-attended on 13 and 31 Oct.

21 Oct. Mother attended, and complained again of feeling tired.

29 Oct. Mother re-attended, and told me that her breasts were 'painful'. No abnormal signs were discovered.

10 Nov. Alma had bronchitis.

24 Nov. Mother complained again of tiredness.

8 Dec. Mother came with Celia and told me that the child's eyes were 'swelling up'. I found no abnormality.

19 Jan. 1959. Mother attended complaining of tiredness.

4 Feb. Alma had conjunctivitis.

12 Feb. Mother brought Alma to surgery and told me that the child had complained of pain in her neck. On examination she was found to have slightly enlarged and tender jugular lymph glands on one side.

5 March. Mother attended complaining of low backache. She had a mild sacroiliac strain.

10 March. Husband attended and complained of 'fluttering in the stomach'. I found no abnormality.

4 April. Husband re-attended.

13 April. Mother re-attended with sacroiliac strain, and she had now become pregnant. She also told me that she was afraid of having cancer.

20 April. Celia had a recurrence of the small anal tear.

Sept. Mother had gastroenteritis.

99

Oct. Mother had a recurrence of the sacroiliac strain.

FAMILY 34

Jan. Husband attended and complained of 'wind'. Further history suggested that he had mild flatulence; I found no abnormal signs. (The husband and wife had recently had medical investigations, and the results were within normal limits).

Feb. Husband had a head cold and re-attended twice.

March. Husband re-attended and complained of feeling dizzy. No abnormalities were found.

March. Four days later. Wife attended and told me that she was afraid that she might have 'cancer'. I found nothing abnormal on examining her.

2 April. Husband attended complaining that he felt 'run down'. No abnormalities were discovered.

29 April. Wife re-attended still with cancer phobia.

26 June. Husband attended again with a head cold.

28 June. Wife attended. She had a mild gastritis and other symptoms which appeared to be functional.

31 July. Wife attended complaining of pruritus vulvae. There were no abnormal signs.

21 Aug. Wife re-attended. The pruritus had not improved; in view of my knowledge of the patient I withheld routine investigations and gave her sedatives as symptomatic treatment.

27 Aug. Wife came with daughter, and told me that the girl had been 'off-colour'. I found no abnormal signs; and asked her to come back if the girl was not better within a short time.

The wife re-attended twice with vaginal pruritus.

20 Sept. Wife attended and told me that she was depressed; her husband had been unfaithful. This she had found out one month previously.

7 Oct. Wife re-attended and said that she could not sleep.

11 Oct. Wife came with daughter and complained that the child was 'off-colour' again.

24 Oct. Wife attended, complaining of depression. She told me that her husband was going to leave her to live with the other woman.

27 Oct. Husband came to see me about a tender spot on his neck. He also said that his 'nerves were bad' and he had 'indigestion'. The tenderness was due to a slightly enlarged jugular lymph gland. He had no other abnormality.

(He left his wife a few days later and returned to her early in February.)

29 Nov. Wife had a mild upper respiratory tract infection.

16 Feb. Husband attended shortly after his return. He had a mild upper respiratory tract infection, and other symptoms which I thought were functional in origin.

March. Wife attended; she had a trichomonas vaginitis.

May. Husband attended with vague abdominal pains. I found no abnormality on examination.

2 June. Husband attended, complaining of pain in his calves on walking which was relieved by rest. The popliteal pulses were present, but the tibial pulses were not palpable.

18 June. Wife attended, and told me that she was depressed; there had again been marital discord.

July. Wife re-attended, still complaining of depression.

Oct. Wife attended. She said that she was worried and told me that her husband and daughter did not get on well with each other.

5 Nov. Husband attended complaining of pain in his chest. The description of the pain was vague. It was not related to exertion and there were no relieving or aggravating factors. No abnormality was discovered on examination.

19 Nov. Wife attended with acne rosacea which had become more conspicuous.

Dec. Husband attended with pain on defaecation; he had a few small ulcers of the anal mucosa.

APPENDIX III

Tables 16 to 20

This appendix contains tables showing the age and sex distribution of the patients in the samples investigated and two other tables on which histograms were based.

TABLE 16 FAMILY SIZE IN GROUPS A AND B

Number of members	2	3	4	5	6	7	8	9	*Total*
Group A ('neurotic families')	38	25	19	7	3	4	0	1	97
Group B ('non-neurotic families')	28	29	22	17	5	1	0	1	103
Total	66	54	41	24	8	5	0	2	200

TABLE 17 AGE DISTRIBUTION OF PARENTS, 'HUSBANDS AND WIVES' (CHILDLESS OR CHILDREN LIVE AWAY), AND OTHERS (GRANDPARENTS, IN-LAWS, ETC.)

	Group A								
Age	10-	20-	30-	40-	50-	60-	70-	80-	*Total*
Mothers	—	9	28	17	9	2	3	1	69
Fathers	—	2	19	20	13	1	1	1	57
'Husbands'	—	1	3	2	7	7	—	—	20
'Wives'	—	1	4	0	9	6	—	—	20
Others	—	1	—	2	4	4	5	—	16
Total	—	14	54	41	42	20	9	2	182

Group B

Age	10-	20-	30-	40-	50-	60-	70-	80-	*Total*
Mothers	—	12	33	20	10	—	—	—	75
Fathers	—	4	26	26	10	3	—	—	69
'Husbands'	—	—	4	4	5	3	2	—	18
'Wives'	—	1	5	1	7	2	2	—	18
Others	7	2	—	3	1	5	2	—	20
Total	7	19	68	54	33	13	6	—	200

TABLE 18 AGE DISTRIBUTION
OF 'CHILDREN'

Group A

Age	0-	5-	10-	15-	20-	25-	*Total*
Girls	11	13	20	16	5	7	72
Boys	14	17	18	9	2	3	63
Total	25	30	38	25	7	10	135

Group B

Age	0-	5-	10-	15-	20-	25-	*Total*
Girls	19	23	23	15	3	1	84
Boys	18	20	19	12	8	1	78
Total	37	43	42	27	11	2	162

TABLE 19 AGE DISTRIBUTION OF 'NEUROTIC' PATIENTS
AND OTHERS IN GROUPS A1 AND B1

	Age	0-	10-	20-	30-	40-	50-	60-	70-	80-	*Total*
Fe-	'neurotic'										
male	patients	0	10	14	30	18	18	9	4	—	103
A1	Relatives	25	26	7	7	1	—	—	3	1	70
	Total	25	36	21	37	19	18	9	7	1	173
Male	'neurotic'										
A1	patients	4	1	4	14	10	6	4	1	—	44
	Relatives	28	28	3	9	14	20	8	1	1	112
	Total	32	29	7	23	24	26	12	2	1	156
B1	Female	41	39	18	36	21	17	4	4	0	180
	Male	36	35	14	29	32	16	9	2	0	173
	Total	77	74	32	65	53	33	13	6	—	353

TABLE 20 NUMBER OF PATIENTS HAVING CONSULTED AT LEAST ONCE IN TWO YEARS

				Group A1					
Family size	2	3	4	5	6	7	8	9	*Total*
Consulting patients	73	64	63	38	15	24	0	7	284
Non-consulting patients	5	11	13	7	3	4	0	2	45
Total	78	75	76	45	18	28	0	9	329
				Group B1					
Family size	2	3	4	5	6	7	8	9	*Total*
Consulting patients	37	50	57	57	22	5	0	5	233
Non-consulting patients	17	34	27	28	8	2	0	4	120
Total	54	84	84	85	30	7	0	9	353

Statistical Report on the Incidence of 'Paired Consultations'[1]

M. C. K. TWEEDIE AND B. SELBY

Statistical tests showed that nearly all, or perhaps all, of the increase in number of the remaining pairs in Group A was due to members of this group tending to consult considerably more often than members of Group B as can be seen in Table 21 (ignoring family size).

TABLE 21 FREQUENCY OF CONSULTATIONS IN GROUPS A AND B

Number of consultations	0-5	6-10	11-15	16-
Frequency in Group A	14	23	20	40
Frequency in Group B	53	33	11	6

In order to determine whether or not there existed a pairing effect in Group A, an investigation was made of the relationship between the actual number of pairs and the maximum number of pairs which would be possible with the given

[1] An extract from this report has been presented in Chapter 4.

number of consultations made by the members of a particular family. The relationship tended to be nearly the same for both groups with families of equal size, and did not depend greatly on size of family over the range 2-4.

There was however a moderately strong indication, probably significant (if an exact test were made) at the usual conventional 5 per cent level, of a difference between Groups A and B in families of size 2. Group A give slightly more pairs than Group B than could be easily accounted for by the greater number of consultations made by 'A' patients.

The comparison between the two groups was made on the basis of theoretical considerations which indicated that, if the consultations were more or less randomly distributed, the number of pairs from a given family would tend to be a fraction (α, say) of the maximum possible number of pairs. The maximum possible number of pairs was computed by a simple algebraic formula. As a numerical example, consider a family of 3 persons with 4, 3, and 4 consultations. The maximum possible number of pairs $= 4 \times 3 + 4 \times 4 + 3 \times 4 = 40$, whereas a family of equal size with an equal total number of consultations but in the pattern 7, 2, 2, produced $7 \times 2 + 7 \times 2 + 2 \times 2 = 32$ pairs at most.

REFERENCES

APLEY, J. (1958). Common denominators in the recurrent pains of childhood. *Proc. Roy. Soc. Med.* **51,** 1023.

APLEY, J. (1959). *The child with abdominal pains.* Oxford: Blackwell.

BACKET, E. M., SHAW, M. A. & EVANS, J. G. G. (1953). Studies of a general practice. Patients' needs and doctors' services. *Proc. Roy. Soc. Med.* **46,** 707.

BALINT, M. (1957) *The doctor, his patient and the illness.* London: Pitman.

BALINT, M. *et al.* (1960) Personal communication.

BOWLBY, J. (1952). *Maternal care and mental health.* W. H. O. Geneva.

BUCK, C. W. & LAUGHTON, K. B. (1959). Family patterns of illness. The effect of psychoneurosis in the parent upon the illness of the child. *Acta Psychol. & Neurol. Scand.* **34,** 165.

BUCK, C. W. (1962). Personal communication.

COOLRIDGE, J. C. (1956). Asthma in mother and child. *Amer. J. Orthopsychiat.* **26,** 165.

COWIE, V. (1961). Children of psychotics. A controlled study. *Proc. Roy. Soc. Med.* **8,** 54.

DOWNES, J. & SIMON, K. (1953). Characteristics of psychoneurotic patients and their families as revealed in a general morbidity study. *Psychosom. Med.* **15,** 463.

FRY, J. (1954). The psychoneurotic in general practice. *Med. World,* **80,** 6.

FRY, J. (1957). Five years in general practice. A study in simple epidemiology. *Brit. med. J.* **2,** 1453.

GREGORY, I. (1959). Husbands and wives admitted to mental hospitals. *J. ment. Sci.* **105,** 457.

HOPKINS, P. (1959). Health and happiness and the family. *Brit. J. clin. Pract.* **13,** 311.

References

HUNTER, R. A. & ROSS, I. P. (1960) Psychotherapy in migraine. *Brit. med. J.* **1,** 1084.

KELLNER, R. (1962). The premenstrual tension syndrome. Attendances in a general practice. (Forthcoming).

KESSEL, W. I. N. (1960). Psychiatric morbidity in a London general practice. *Brit. J. prev. soc. med.* **14,** 16.

LOGAN, W. P. D. & CUSHION, A. A. (1958). *Morbidity statistics from general practice.* Volume 1 (General). Studies on medical population subjects No. 14. London: H.M.S.O.

MEYER, R. J. & HAGGERTY, R. J. (1962). Streptococcal infection in families. Factors altering individual susceptibility. *Pediatrics* **29,** 539.

MURSTEIN, B. I. (1960). The effects of long-term illness of children on the emotional adjustment of parents. *Child Developm.* **31,** 157.

PASMORE, H. S. (1959). Psychiatry in general practice. *Brit. J. clin. Pract.* **13,** 70.

PAULET, J. D. (1956). Neurotic ill health. A study in general practice. *Lancet* **2,** 37.

PEMBERTON, J. (1949). Illness in general practice. *Brit. med. J.* **1,** 306.

PENROSE, L. S. (1944). Mental illness in husband and wife. A contribution to the study of assortative mating in man. *Psychiat. Quart. Suppt.* **18,** 161.

POST, F. & WARDLE, J. (1962). Family neurosis and family psychosis. A review of the problem. *J. ment. Sci.* **108,** 147.

POUGHER, J. C. E. (1955). Neurosis in general practice. *Brit. med. J.* **2,** 409.

Psychological medicine in general practice. (1958). A report prepared by a working party of the Council of the College of General Practitioners. *Brit. med. J.* **2,** 585.

REES, L. (1953). Psychosomatic aspects of the premenstrual tension syndrome. *J. ment. Sci.* **99,** 62.

RUTTER, M. L. (1962). *Illness in parents and children.* (Forthcoming).

SIRCUS, W. (1959). The management of recurrent aphtous stomatitis. *Brit. med. J.* **2,** 804.

SLATER, E. & WOODSIDE, M. (1951). *Patterns of Marriage.* London: Cassell.

WATTS, C. A. H. (1956). The incidence and prognosis of endogenous depression. *Brit. med. J.* **1,** 1392.

WOLFF, H. G. (1952) Stress and disease. Springfield, Ill.: C. C. Thomas.

INDEX

accident, road, 10
acne rosacea, 21
acne vulgaris, 9
acrocyanosis, 91
age distribution
adults, 102
children, 103
in families, 58
neurotic patients, 103
agoraphobia, 93
anaemia, hypochromic, 37, 96
anal mucosa
tears, 98, 99
ulcers, 101
ankle, inversion, 95
anxiety symptoms, 15, 22, 23, 28, 31, 33, 37, 92, 97
aphthous stomatitis, 30
arthrotomy, exploratory, 90
asthma, 21, 56, 88
doubtful interaction, 50
patients and relatives with neurotic symptoms, 66
attendance charts, description, 81
attendances
family rates, 55, 62
high, 66
consultations and re-visits, 67
paired, 60
see also visits

attenders
average, 22
frequent, 35, 85
rare, 7
reasons, 55

bed-wetting, 85, 93
behaviour disorder, 37, 53
blood loss, menstrual, excessive, 98
bolus hystericus, 94, 95
breast, carcinoma, 20, 49
bronchitis, 9, 10, 14, 23, 25, 31, 33, 89, 93, 95, 97, 98, 99
bursa, olecranon, distension, 12

cancer phobia, 99, 100
cellulitis, 31, 94
chest pain, 37, 92, 94, 97, 98, 101
children
effect of neuroses on, 53, 77
and parents, interaction, 52
clusters, 42, and *passim*
incidence, apparent causes, 60, 61
coincidence
and infection, 42
pairing and clustering, 48, 49, 61
conjunctivitis, 21, 99
constipation, 34